Panic Anxiety and Its Treatments

Panic Anxiety and Its Treatments

Report of the World Psychiatric Association
Presidential Educational Program Task Force
Jorge Alberto Costa e Silva, M.D., President

Edited by

Gerald L. Klerman, M.D.
Robert M. A. Hirschfeld, M.D.
Myrna M. Weissman, Ph.D.
Yves Pelicier, M.D.
James C. Ballenger, M.D.
Jorge Alberto Costa e Silva, M.D.
Lewis L. Judd, M.D.
Martin B. Keller, M.D.

Prepared by

Members of the Task Force on
Panic Anxiety and Its Treatments

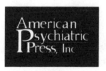

Washington, DC
London, England

Note: The authors have worked to ensure that all information in this book concerning drug dosages, schedules, and routes of administration is accurate as of the time of publication and consistent with standards set by the U.S. Food and Drug Administration and the general medical community. As medical research and practice advance, however, therapeutic standards may change. For this reason and because human and mechanical errors sometimes occur, we recommend that readers follow the advice of a physician who is directly involved in their care or the care of a member of their family.

Books published by the American Psychiatric Press, Inc., represent the views and opinions of the individual authors and do not necessarily represent the policies and opinions of the Press or the American Psychiatric Association.

Copyright © 1993 World Psychiatric Association
ALL RIGHTS RESERVED
Manufactured in the United States of America on acid-free paper
96 95 94 93   4 3 2 1
First Edition

American Psychiatric Press, Inc.
1400 K Street, N.W., Washington, DC   20005

Library of Congress Cataloging-in-Publication Data
Panic anxiety and its treatments : report of the World Psychiatric
  Association Presidential Educational Task Force / edited by Gerald
  L. Klerman . . . [et al.] ; prepared by members of the Task Force—
  Panic Anxiety and Its Treatments. — 1st ed.
     p.   cm.
  At head of title: World Psychiatric Association, American
Psychiatric Press.
  Includes bibliographical references and index.
  ISBN 0-88048-684-8 (alk. paper)
  1. Panic disorders.   I. Klerman, Gerald L., 1928–1992.   II. World
Psychiatric Association.   Presidential Educational Task Force.
III. World Psychiatric Association.   Task Force—Panic Anxiety and
Its Treatments.
  [DNLM: 1. Panic Disorder. 2. Phobic Disorders.   WM 172 P1924
1993]
RC535.P354 1993
616.85′223—dc20
DNLM/DLC
for Library of Congress   93-16381
                                                                          CIP

British Library Cataloguing in Publication Data
A CIP record is available from the British Library.

Dedication to
Gerald L. Klerman, M.D.

This book is dedicated to Gerald L. Klerman, M.D., the lead author, who died April 3, 1992, before the final version had been completed. In 1991, when Gerry was invited by Jorge Alberto Costa e Silva, M.D., President of the World Psychiatric Association, to chair this project, he undertook it with great enthusiasm. He felt that sufficient empirical information on many aspects of panic disorder had become available over the past decade and that a compilation of this information was timely and of public health importance to the world.

Gerry assembled an international group of experts to advise and assist. He prepared nearly 80 pages for the first meeting of experts held in Sonesta Beach, Florida, in May 1991. Over the next months with the experts' assistance, he began to fill in the missing parts. When the second meeting of advisers was held in November 1991 in Acapulco, Mexico, in conjunction with the Mexican Psychiatric Association meeting, Gerry was too ill to travel. The group met in Mexico, and Gerry participated all day via teleconference. Minutes were taken by his assistant, Mrs. Marlene Carlson. Gerry's long-term colleague, Robert Hirschfeld, M.D., chaired the Mexican part of the telephone conference. Gerry was undaunted by the periodic breaks in the telephone hookup that day or his waning physical health. He remained enthusiastic and committed to completing the project. When he died, the second draft of the volume was ready for his revision.

The Scientific Editorial Group met after Gerry's death in May 1992 in Washington, DC, in conjunction with the American Psychiatric Association annual meeting to decide how to best complete the project. Gerry's good friends and scientific colleagues from all over the world unselfishly responded to requests for information to complete missing portions, provide updates, and check material. Redundancies and changes in the style of writing are a reflection of the effort of many people to complete this work in the absence of Gerry's integrating ability.

This volume and context of its process is a true reflection of Gerry the man and the scientist. He was committed to scientific excellence that knew neither ideologic nor international bounds. He was able to get the best product from the best people and select among them wisely. His work, despite considerable physical difficulties, was not selfless nor sacrificial, but came from the commitment to the task and a pleasure of the process, people, and product.

Myrna M. Weissman (Klerman), Ph.D.
New York, New York
January 5, 1993

Acknowledgments

The authors would like to express their thanks and appreciation to Mrs. Marlene Carlson, Ms. Barbara Schwedel, and Ms. Kathleen Talbot, whose assistance in the preparation of this book was invaluable.

We wish to acknowledge and thank the following people, who contributed material that has been incorporated into this volume:

Kenneth Kendler, M.D.
Professor of Psychiatry
Department of Psychiatry
Medical College of Virginia
Richmond, Virginia

Matig Mavissakalian, M.D.
Professor of Psychiatry
Director, Phobia and Anxiety Clinic
Ohio State University College of Medicine
Columbus, Ohio

Contents

Dedication to Gerald L. Klerman, M.D. v

Acknowledgments vii

Members of the World Psychiatric Association
    Presidential Educational Program Task Force xiii

Preface xvii

1 Introduction 1

2 Panic Anxiety and Panic Disorder 3
    Clinical and Diagnostic Features 4
        Panic Anxiety 6
        Panic Attacks 7
        Limited Symptom Attacks 7
        Panic Disorder 8
        Nonfearful Panic Disorder 9
        Diagnostic Issues in the DSM and the ICD 10
        Clinical Features 13
    Clinical Assessment 14
        Assessment 14
        Differential Diagnosis 15
        Psychiatric Disorders 15
        Medical Disorders 16
    Interface With General Medicine 18
        Help-Seeking and Somatization 18
        Misdiagnosis and Undertreatment 19
    Epidemiology and Familial Risk 21
        Rates (Prevalence) 21

Risk Factors 22
Family History as a Risk Factor 22
Cross-National and Cross-Cultural Considerations 23
Uncomplicated and Comorbid Panic Disorder 24
Uncomplicated Panic Disorder 24
Comorbidity With Agoraphobia 25
Comorbidity With Other Anxiety Disorders. 26
Comorbidity With Depression 27
Comorbidity With Personality Disorders 28
Comorbidity With Alcoholism 28
Comorbidity With Medical Conditions. 29
Clinical Course and Follow-Up. 30
Medical Morbidity and Mortality 34
Suicide Attempts and Deaths 35
Quality of Life. 36

3 The Origins of Panic Disorder: Etiology and Pathogenesis . . 39
Etiology 39
Genetics and Familial Factors. 40
Psychological Theories: Psychodynamic and
    Psychoanalytic Theories. 42
Psychological Theories: Learning and Behavior Theories . 43
Psychological Theories: Cognitive Theory. 44
Developmental Theories: Childhood Separation Anxiety . . 45
Developmental Theories: Childhood Behavioral Inhibition 45
Developmental Theories: Parental Child-Rearing
    Attitudes and Behavior. 46
Conclusion. 46
Pathogenesis and Pathophysiology: Experimental Models
and Biological Theories. 47
Provocation and Challenge Studies 47
Neuroendocrine and Other Biological Markers 48
Animal Models of Anxiety and Arousal States. 48
Functional Brain Imaging Studies. 48
Nocturnal Panic Attacks 49
Neurochemical and Neurotransmitter Theories. 49
Panic Disorder as a Variant of a Convulsive Disorder . . . 52
A Current Working Hypothesis of Panic Disorder. 52
Pathogenesis and Pathophysiology: Psychological and
Psychosocial Theories. 53

Life Events as Precipitants 53
Predisposing Factors in Adolescent and Adult Personality . 54

4 Validity of Panic Disorder as a Nosological Entity 57
Clinical Description of Panic Disorder 58
Laboratory Studies. 58
Delimitation From Other Disorders 59
Follow-Up Studies 60
Family Studies and Twin Studies 60

5 Treatments for Panic Anxiety: Research Findings 61
General Considerations 61
Psychopharmacological Treatments 61
    Historical Background. 61
    Monoamine Oxidase Inhibitors 65
    Tricyclic Antidepressants 66
        General Considerations. 66
        Imipramine 66
        Clomipramine 68
        Adverse Effects of Tricyclic Antidepressants 69
        Clinical Issues. 70
        Dose During Long-Term Treatment 70
    Benzodiazepines 71
        General Considerations 71
        Alprazolam. 73
        Other Benzodiazepines. 76
        Adverse Effects. 76
        Abuse Potential. 76
        Effect of Comorbidity With Substance Abuse 77
        Dependence. 77
        Clinical Discontinuation Reactions 78
        Rebound 79
        Factors Influencing Benzodiazepine
          Withdrawal in Panic Disorder Patients 79
    Serotonin Reuptake Blocking Agents. 81
    Depression and Psychopharmacological Treatment Response 83
    Comparative Psychopharmacological Studies 84
    Long-Term Psychopharmacological Treatment
      of Panic Disorder 84
        Tricyclic Antidepressants in Long-Term Treatment . . . 86

    Alprazolam and Other Benzodiazepines 87
  Psychological Treatments. 89
    General Considerations 89
    Psychoanalysis and Psychoanalytic-Oriented Therapy . . . 89
    Exposure-Based Therapy. 90
    Relaxation Training. 92
    Cognitive-Behavioral Treatments 93
    Comparative Outcome Studies of Psychosocial
      Treatments 95
    Long-Term Psychological Treatments 98
  Comparative Studies of Psychopharmacological and
  Psychological Treatments 100
  Combined Psychological and Psychopharmacological
  Treatment 103
  Conclusions. 107

6 Clinical Practice Patterns for Panic Disorder. 109
  Patterns of Prescription and Use of Antipanic Medications . . 109
    General Patterns of Use of Benzodiazepines. 110
    Panic Disorder 110
    Treatment Considerations in Clinical Practice. 111

7 Summary, Conclusions, and Recommendations 113
  Summary of Findings 113
  Implications and Guidelines for Clinical Practice 114
  Future Research 115

References 119

Selected Readings 139

Index 151

World Psychiatric Association Presidential Educational Program Task Force on Panic Anxiety and Its Treatments

Chairman: April 1991—April 1992

Gerald L. Klerman, M.D.
Professor and Associate Chairman for Research, Department of Psychiatry, Cornell University Medical College, New York, New York

Chairman: April 1992—Present

** **Robert M. A. Hirschfeld, M.D.**
Professor and Chairman, Department of Psychiatry and Behavioral Sciences, University of Texas Medical Branch, Galveston, Texas

Co-Chairs

* **Professor Yves Pelicier**
Professeur de Psychiatrie, Hôpital Necker-Enfants Malades, Consultations de Psychiatrie et de Psychologie, Clinique des Adultes, Paris, France

* **Myrna M. Weissman, Ph.D.**
Professor, College of Physicians and Surgeons, Columbia University; Chief, Division of Clinical and Genetic Epidemiology, New York State Psychiatric Institute, New York, New York

---

* Members of the Editorial Committee

Members

Kalle Achte, M.D.
Professor and Chairman, Department of Psychiatry, University of
Helsinki, Helsinki, Finland

Christer Allgulander, M.D.
Associate Professor of Psychiatry and Senior Lecturer, Huddinge
University Hospital, Huddinge, Sweden

* **James C. Ballenger, M.D.**
Chairman, Department of Psychiatry and Behavioral Sciences,
Medical University of South Carolina College of Medicine,
Charleston, South Carolina

Mitchell B. Balter, Ph.D.
Adjunct Professor, Department of Pharmacology and Experimental
Therapeutics, Tufts University School of Medicine, Boston,
Massachusetts; Director, Public Health Research Center,
Washington, DC

David H. Barlow, Ph.D.
Distinguished Professor of Psychology, Department of Psychology,
State University of New York at Albany, Albany, New York

* **Jorge Alberto Costa e Silva, M.D.**
President, World Psychiatric Association, Rio de Janeiro, Brazil

George C. Curtis, M.D.
Professor of Psychiatry, Department of Psychiatry, Director, Anxiety
Disorders Program, University of Michigan, Ann Arbor, Michigan

Juan Ramon de la Fuente, M.D.
Dean of the Faculty of Medicine, National University of Mexico,
School of Medicine, Mexico City, Mexico

Michael G. Gelder, M.D.
Professor of Psychiatry, University of Oxford School of Medicine,
Oxford, England

* Lewis L. Judd, M.D.
Professor and Chairman, Department of Psychiatry, University of
California, San Diego, School of Medicine, La Jolla, California

Wayne Katon, M.D.
Professor of Psychiatry, Department of Psychiatry, and Chief,
Division of Consultation-Liaison Psychiatry, University of
Washington Medical School, Seattle, Washington

Heinz Katschnig, M.D.
Allgemeines Krankenhaus Der Stadt Wien, Psychiatrische
Universitatsklinik, Vienna, Austria

* Martin B. Keller, M.D.
Professor and Chairman, Department of Psychiatry and Human
Behavior, Brown University Program in Medicine, Butler Hospital,
Providence, Rhode Island

Juan E. Mezzich, M.D., Ph.D.
Professor of Psychiatry and Epidemiology, Department of
Psychiatry, University of Pittsburgh, Pittsburgh, Pennsylvania

Masahisa Nishizono, M.D.
Professor and Chairman, Department of Psychiatry, School of
Medicine, Fukuoka University, Fukuoka, Japan

Russell Noyes, M.D.
Professor of Psychiatry, University of Iowa College of Medicine, Iowa
City, Iowa

Jan-Otto Ottosson, M.D.
Professor of Psychiatry, University of Gothenburg, Gothenburg,
Sweden

Robert F. Prien, Ph.D.
Director, Clinical Psychopharmacology, Division of Clinical
Research, National Institute of Mental Health, Rockville, Maryland

Robert G. Priest, M.D.
Professor, Academic Department of Psychiatry, St. Mary's Hospital
Medical School, London, England

Karl Rickels, M.D.
Stuart and Emily B. H. Mudd Professor of Human Behavior and
Professor of Psychiatry, Hospital of the University of Pennsylvania,
Philadelphia, Pennsylvania

E. H. Uhlenhuth, M.D.
Professor and Vice Chairman for Education, Department of
Psychiatry, University of New Mexico, Albuquerque, New Mexico

Preface

In 1991, as part of his presidency of the World Psychiatric Association, Professor Dr. Jorge Alberto Costa e Silva initiated a new program of Presidential educational projects. He felt that the first of these projects should be a task force to assess the status of panic anxiety and its treatments.

This book is a report of the Task Force. In it, we review the clinical and epidemiologic findings regarding panic anxiety, particularly as to the validity of the diagnostic concepts, the evidence for efficacy and safety of current treatments, the available knowledge regarding current clinical practices in relation to research findings and public health needs, and the implication of these findings for clinical practice and public policy. We identify areas for future research and then make recommendations to the World Psychiatric Association regarding future educational research programs.

1   Introduction

The clinical phenomenology of panic disorder and agoraphobia has been part of the literature for more than 100 years. However, official attention to these problems has been very recent. For example, panic disorder has been included in the *Diagnostic and Statistical Manual of Mental Disorders* of the American Psychiatric Association only since 1980 and did not appear in the *International Classification of Diseases* of the World Health Organization, the official psychiatric nomenclature of the world, until the recently published 10th revision.

Considerable controversies have arisen about panic anxiety and its treatments. Is panic a separate and distinct diagnosis or an extreme form of phobia? Is it a transient, mild response to everyday stressors or an episodic or chronic illness with substantial morbidity? What is the place of pharmacological, behavioral, or cognitive treatment?

The accumulation of empirical evidence in support of more precise understanding, accurate diagnosis, and effective treatments of panic disorder has proceeded at a very rapid pace during the past decade. This remarkable scientific progress, coupled with the many controversies, has provided the basis for two landmark initiatives for panic disorders in the United States, which occurred in the fall of 1991. The National Institutes of Health (NIH), in cooperation with the National Institute of Mental Health (NIMH), held a Consensus Development Conference on the Treatment of Panic Disorder. The NIMH has established a panic education and prevention program directed at both the public and mental health professionals. Its purpose is to increase the awareness of panic disorder and to actively encourage those with this disorder to seek treatment.

In light of these developments, the World Psychiatric Association has established a Task Force on Panic Anxiety and Its Treatments. A major product of the task force is this volume, which summarizes the current scientific knowledge on panic disorder. It begins with a presentation of the important clinical and diagnostic features of panic anxiety that includes assessment, interface with general medicine, epidemiology and comorbidity, clinical course, and the effect on quality of life.

The next chapter discusses what is known about the causes of panic anxiety—both biological and psychological theories and evidence. Evidence supporting the validity of panic disorder as a diagnostic entity is also included.

A thorough presentation of the treatments for panic anxiety follows. Information about the various pharmacotherapies and psychotherapies is reviewed, including evidence for efficacy, indications, and side effects. Issues related to long-term treatment are addressed. Finally, there is a chapter on combined pharmacological and psychotherapeutic treatments. The last substantive chapter describes patterns of current drug prescriptions and usages around the world.

The volume concludes with recommendations for the future.

2   Panic Anxiety and Panic Disorder

Although descriptions of clinical conditions that today would be labeled panic disorder can be found in Elizabethan and Victorian writings, modern scientific interest in the disorder is only a few decades old. In those few decades, there has been considerable research on the clinical, epidemiological, biological, and psychological aspects of panic disorder. The fundamental rationale for this attention rests on the growing evidence that panic disorder is a serious psychopathological condition associated with high prevalence, tendencies toward chronicity and recurrence over time, significant impairment in quality of life and social functioning, increased morbidity and mortality from medical illness, and suicide. One practical yield from this research has been psychopharmacological and psychological treatments that are now widely available.

The purpose of this chapter is to describe the clinical condition of panic disorder and what happens to persons with the disorder. It begins with an overview of the development of the concept of panic disorder, refinements in its clinical description, and its acceptance into the official nomenclature. This chapter then reviews the clinical assessment of persons with panic symptoms, including differential diagnosis. Because many persons with panic symptoms seek help from primary care physicians or nonpsychiatric specialists and because panic disorder appears to have a complex interaction with medical illness—sometimes triggering it, sometimes mimicking it, and sometimes resulting from it (Rogers et al. 1991)—the interface between panic disorder and general medicine is addressed in depth in this chapter. It also reviews the epidemiology of panic disorder, its comorbidity with both psychiatric and medical disorders, and its clinical course and follow-up. Finally, evidence that the consequences of panic disorder are serious, particularly with respect to morbidity, mortality, and quality of life, is summarized.

Clinical and Diagnostic Features

Clinical descriptions of the condition that we today consider panic disorder were frequent in the 19th century. For example, the German psychiatrist Westphal (1872) published his observations on four patients with agoraphobia that we now recognize as a description of the classic symptoms of the syndrome. He described in detail the rapid development of phobic fears of being in wide, open spaces and fears of other public places, such as certain streets or theaters, and characterized the syndrome as initially appearing suddenly and "out of the blue" with no apparent reason. He also described the anticipatory anxiety of the patients when they knew they had to enter one of these phobic situations or even when they were thinking about that possibility. Although Westphal did not emphasize panic attacks, he gave clear and surprisingly modern descriptions of sudden panic attacks occurring both spontaneously and in phobic situations.

At about the same time, Dr. Jacob DaCosta (1871) vividly described panic attacks on the basis of his observations of soldiers in the American Civil War and his readings of other historians of military medicine.

A turning point in the descriptive nosology of panic disorder came in 1894 with Freud's use of the term "anxiety neurosis" for the first time and his proposal of the separation of anxiety neurosis from neurasthenia. Freud also provided a clinical description of two types of anxiety that today would be labeled panic attacks and generalized anxiety. He later described panic attacks as "[when] the connection between anxiety and a threatening danger is completely lost to view . . . spontaneous attacks . . . represented by intensely developed symptoms . . . tremor, vertigo, palpitations of the heart" (Freud 1917/1963). Freud also noted the comorbidity of panic disorder with depression and the high degree of associated avoidance behavior and social disability.

The literature on anxiety grew gradually between World Wars I and II. "Cardiac neuroses" and "soldier's heart" figured prominently in World War I military psychiatry. One important group of early studies was conducted by cardiologists at the Massachusetts General Hospital under the leadership of Paul Dudley White. They collected the data on a large number of patients referred to them for diagnostic evaluation and identified a group of patients who, they concluded, did not have organic heart disease but did have a functional disorder that they diagnosed as "neurocirculatory asthenia." They conducted a number of studies on this diagnostic group, including important follow-up studies, that indicated that the initial disorder remained stable and that the patients did not later acquire structural heart disease. Also at Massachusetts General Hospital, a group of neuropsychiatrists under the leadership of Mandell Cohen gave careful clinical descriptions of what they labeled "anxiety neurosis" but what today we would consider panic disorder. Neurocirculatory asthenia was described during World War II. In the postwar period, Cohen reported the first family study on the disorder, and the clinical syndrome became further delineated. In Great Britain, Roth (1960) described phobic depersonalization, a syndrome similar to panic disorder.

In the 1950s and 1960s, extensive clinical investigations were conducted on a variety of psychopharmacological treatments for panic disorder, including barbiturates, phenothiazines, meprobamate, beta-adrenergic blocking agents, and several nonbarbiturate sedatives. Those treatments were almost uniformly found to be ineffective. In the 1960s, two parallel discoveries in psychopharmacology laid the groundwork for effective treatment of patients with panic disorder: 1) the demonstration of the efficacy of monoamine oxidase inhibitors (MAOIs) for "atypical depression" and "phobic anxiety," first described in Great Britain (Kelly et al. 1970; Sargant and Dally 1962); and 2) the demonstration of the efficacy of tricyclic antidepressants (TCAs), which was first reported in the United States (Fink et al. 1965; Klein 1964; Klein and Fink 1962).

Another line of investigation was initiated by Pitts and McClure (1967), who studied the effects of infused lactate. They observed that persons with a history of anxiety neurosis (i.e., panic disorder) were prone to experience episodes similar to panic attacks during the infusion of sodium lactate. The research of Pitts and McClure provided a foundation for more recent investigations of the experimental induction of panic attacks in the laboratory with a variety of provocative agents, including lactate (Klein 1981), caffeine (Uhde et al. 1985), yohimbine (Charney et al. 1987; Uhde et al. 1985), and carbon dioxide (van den Hout and Griez 1982).

Clinical, biological, and epidemiological research on panic disorder during this period was greatly enhanced by advances in general psychopathology, particularly the development of operational diagnostic criteria, a process for the validation of diagnostic algorithms, and structured interviews. In the United States, diagnostic algorithms were first provided in the Renard Washington University Criteria

(Feighner et al. 1972; L. N. Robins et al. 1977) and were later expanded into the Research Diagnostic Criteria (RDC; Spitzer et al.
1978). The RDC established a set of diagnostic criteria for 22 selected
disorders, including panic disorders, and provided a framework for
similar diagnostic criteria in an expanded list of disorders in the *Diagnostic and Statistical Manual of Mental Disorders, Third Edition*
(DSM-III; American Psychiatric Association [APA] 1980).

Structured diagnostic interviews were developed that allowed for
systematic coverage of a range of past and current psychopathology
in a manner that increases the reliability and comprehensiveness of
the information generated (Endicott and Spitzer 1978; Wing et al.
1974).

The multiple lines of investigation reached their culmination in
1980 with the publication of the DSM-III, which, among other innova-
tions, gave official recognition to panic disorder as a diagnostic category. The DSM-III also developed diagnostic criteria into an
algorithm, the basic structure of which was only partially modified by
the *Diagnostic and Statistical Manual of Mental Disorders, Third Edition, Revised* (DSM-III-R; APA 1987).

The category "Panic Disorder" appears in the draft for the 10th revision of the *International Classification of Diseases* (ICD-10; World
Health Organization 1990). Although the DSM-III concepts of differ-
entiated anxiety disorders and of panic disorder as a separate condition have gained widespread acceptance, this acceptance has not been
universal. There are significant areas of disagreement and controversy, which are discussed in greater detail in Chapter 4.

Familiarity with several basic concepts pertinent to panic disorder
is essential to a discussion of the disorder. Those concepts are briefly
reviewed in the following paragraphs. The information provided is
predominantly from the perspective of the DSM. The specific details of
the definitions given in the DSM have evolved over time, but the broad
concepts underlying them for the most part have been consistent.

Panic Anxiety

Panic anxiety refers to the anxiety symptoms that occur during panic
attacks or limited symptom attacks, described later. There is wide
agreement on the clinical features of panic anxiety. Panic anxiety, in
contrast with generalized anxiety, is characterized by a sudden onset
of distressing body organ symptoms, often accompanied by thoughts of

dread, impending doom, death, and fear of being trapped. The 13 symptoms of panic anxiety in the DSM-III-R are listed in Table 1. The clinical manifestations of panic anxiety, as classified by the DSM-III-R and the ICD-10, are shown in Tables 2 and 3.

Panic Attacks

Panic attacks are sudden, spontaneous episodes accompanied by symptoms such as palpitations, dyspnea, dizziness, and a feeling that death is imminent. To qualify as a panic attack according to the DSM-III-R, at least 4 of the 13 symptoms of panic anxiety must occur during an individual episode. We now know that many persons have panic attacks that do not occur in sufficient frequency to meet all the DSM-III criteria for panic disorder (Klerman et al. 1990; Norton et al. 1992). Moreover, a gradient has been observed: The degree of disability and help-seeking behavior correlates with the number and intensity of attacks (Klerman et al. 1990).

Limited Symptom Attacks

Some persons experience limited symptom attacks, which are episodes of anxiety during which there are fewer than the number of symptoms required to meet the DSM-III criteria for a panic attack (four). An anxiety attack with three or fewer symptoms qualifies as a limited symptom attack.

Table 1. DSM-III-R panic attack symptoms

Shortness of breath (dyspnea) or smothering sensations	Nausea or abdominal distress
	Depersonalization or derealization
Dizziness, unsteady feelings, or faintness	Numbness or tingling sensations (paresthesia)
Palpitations or accelerated heart rate (tachycardia)	Flushes (hot flashes) or chills
Trembling or shaking	Chest pain or discomfort
Sweating	Fear of dying
Choking	Fear of going crazy or doing something uncontrolled

Panic Disorder

Panic disorder is an anxiety disorder characterized by the presence of discrete, unexpected episodes of intense somatic symptoms and, at times, cognitions.

Table 2.   DSM-III-R diagnostic criteria for panic disorder

A. At some time during the disturbance, one or more panic attacks (discrete periods of intense fear or discomfort) have occurred that were unexpected, i.e., did not occur immediately before or on exposure to a situation that almost always caused anxiety, and were not triggered by situations in which the person was the focus of others' attention.

B. Either four attacks, as defined in criterion A, have occurred within a four-week period, or one or more attacks have been followed by a period of at least one month of persistent fear of having another attack.

C. At least four of the following symptoms developed during at least one of the attacks:

  ▼ shortness of breath (dyspnea) or smothering sensations

  ▼ dizziness, unsteady feelings, or faintness

  ▼ palpitations or accelerated heart rate (tachycardia)

  ▼ trembling or shaking

  ▼ sweating

  ▼ choking

  ▼ nausea or abdominal distress

  ▼ depersonalization or derealization

  ▼ numbness or tingling sensations (paresthesia)

  ▼ flushes (hot flashes) or chills

  ▼ chest pain or discomfort

  ▼ fear of dying

  ▼ fear of going crazy or doing something uncontrolled

  Note: Attacks involving ≥ 4 symptoms are panic attacks; attacks involving < 4 symptoms are limited symptom attacks.

D. During at least some of the attacks, at least four of the C symptoms developed suddenly and increased in intensity within 10 minutes of the beginning of the first C symptom noticed in the attack.

E. It cannot be established that an organic factor initiated and maintained the disturbance, such as amphetamine or caffeine intoxication or hyperthyroidism.

Source. American Psychiatric Association 1987.

Table 3. ICD-10 diagnostic criteria for panic disorder

A. At least several severe attacks consisting of autonomic anxiety symptoms should have occurred within about one month:

- ▼ in circumstances without objective danger
- ▼ without confinement to known or predictable situations
- ▼ with relative freedom from anxiety symptoms between attacks (although anticipatory anxiety is common)

B. If any of the phobias is present, panic disorder should not be the main diagnosis

C. If the criteria for a depressive disorder are fulfilled at the same time the criteria for panic disorder are met, panic disorder should not be the main diagnosis

Source. Adapted from World Health Organization 1992 with permission.

In the DSM-III and the DSM-III-R, the panic attack has been conceived as the central symptom of panic disorder with anticipatory anxiety and agoraphobia suggested as sequelae to recurrent panic attacks. In contrast, the ICD-9 (World Health Organization 1977) has positioned anxiety and phobic states as parallel categories.

To meet the DSM-III-R criteria for panic disorder, a person must have had four or more panic attacks within a 4-week period or one attack followed by a month of worry (see Table 2). Each attack must have at least 4 of the 13 symptoms, and at least one of the attacks must have "developed suddenly" (i.e., a "spontaneous attack"). The attacks must not be caused by another disorder or related to the patient being the focus of others' attention.

In the DSM-III-R, panic disorder is subdivided into panic disorder without and with agoraphobia, and the current severity of agoraphobic avoidance is subdivided into mild, moderate, and severe. Additionally, a distinction is made between partial and full remission of agoraphobia.

Nonfearful Panic Disorder

Nonfearful panic disorder has been described (Kushner et al. 1990) as a lactate-sensitive subtype of panic disorder responsive to antipanic medications. Because of the numerous somatic symptoms and a conspicuous absence of a self-report of fear, persons with this disorder are frequently encountered in various medical settings, where they often undergo diagnostic procedures that are complex, unnecessary, or both and receive inadequate treatment. Further studies must be undertaken to understand the relation between classic panic disorder and this uncommon condition.

Diagnostic Issues in the DSM and the ICD

As mentioned previously, the content of this report is based largely on the DSM-III and DSM-III-R descriptions of panic disorder. However, any comprehensive review of panic disorder requires identification of the most important features of those descriptions that are at variance with the previous American description (the DSM-II; APA 1968) and, more important, with the approach of the other major diagnostic system, the ICD, particularly the draft for ICD-10 (World Health Organization 1978, 1990).

The DSM-III and the DSM-III-R represented a major change from the DSM-II. Among the most notable changes were the use of operational diagnostic criteria, the multiaxial classification, and the elimination of the distinction between "neurotic" and "psychotic" disorders. Also, the previous category of "neuroses" underwent differentiation into a number of separate categories, including anxiety disorders, affective (mood) disorders, dissociative disorders, and somatoform disorders.

The overall subject of the successive editions of the DSM is "mental disorders" without the necessary presumption that those disorders are medical illnesses or diseases in the framework of general medicine. The term "disorder" is used throughout DSM-III to avoid some of the uncertainties and controversies associated with previously used terms such as "illness" and "reaction type disease." The term "mental disorders" itself is a subject of some controversy because it is part of the overlap in professional interest between psychology and psychiatry in the domain of psychopathology.

In contrast, the ICD system through ICD-9 continued the classic distinction between the functional states of "psychoses" and "neuroses." There is a great deal of compatibility between the DSM-III-R system and the proposed draft ICD-10 in categories such as "mood disorders" and "anxiety disorders." However, although the ICD-10 includes a category of "panic disorder," it does not place panic disorder in a psychopathogenetic linkage to agoraphobia as does the DSM-III-R.

As revealed in the discussions of comorbidity, critics of the DSM-III-R revisions call attention to epidemiological studies that indicated that there may be significant numbers of persons in the community who report agoraphobic symptoms without a current or past panic disorder or even panic attacks.

There is relatively little disagreement on the clinical criteria for limited symptom attacks and panic attacks, and they are widely used in clinical and research endeavors. What is under discussion is the relation of these clinical phenomena to agoraphobia and other states. Some critics of the DSM-III system question the prominence given to panic anxiety and whether the available empirical evidence is of sufficient strength to justify regarding panic disorder as a separate diagnostic category rather than as a severe form of generalized anxiety. These issues are discussed again as they bear on the validity of panic disorder as an independent diagnostic entity (see Chapter 4).

The DSM-III-R groups a number of distinct conditions within the anxiety disorders (Table 4). The distinction between panic disorder and generalized anxiety disorder is notable. That distinction was not previously made in an official diagnostic system, although it was embodied in the RDC, which were widely accepted in research circles in the United States and parts of western Europe before the publication of the DSM-III.

DSM-III and DSM-III-R conceptualizations of panic disorder have had a major impact on the ICD. Panic disorder appeared in ICD for the first time as a distinct nosological entity when it appeared in ICD-10

Table 4. DSM-III-R classification of anxiety disorders

300.00	Anxiety Disorder Not Otherwise Specified
300.01	Panic Disorder Without Agoraphobia
300.02	Generalized Anxiety Disorder
300.21	Panic Disorder With Agoraphobia
300.22	Agoraphobia Without History of Panic Disorder
300.23	Social Phobia
300.29	Simple Phobia
300.30	Obsessive-Compulsive Disorder (or Obsessive-Compulsive Neurosis)
309.89	Posttraumatic Stress Disorder

Source. American Psychiatric Association 1987.

(Table 5). The 1990 draft of ICD-10 uses the diagnostic term "panic disorder" interchangeably with "episodic paroxysmal anxiety," but the description of panic disorder in the ICD-10 is essentially the same as that in the DSM-III-R. However, the ICD-10 gives diagnostic precedence to one of the "phobic anxiety disorders" if a panic attack occurs in an "established phobic situation." This provision reflects a primarily British conceptualization of panic anxiety as a severe form of phobic anxiety if and when it is experienced in a phobic situation. The ICD-10 diagnosis of panic disorder will, therefore, be restricted to panic attacks that initially and continuously occur unpredictably (spontaneously); if agoraphobia develops, panic attacks occurring in agoraphobic situations will be regarded as manifestations of phobic anxiety, and the diagnosis will then be changed to agoraphobia with panic disorder, provided that the unpredictable panic attacks do not disappear.

Table 5. ICD-10 classification of anxiety disorders

F40	**Phobic Anxiety Disorders**	
	F40.0	Agoraphobia
		F40.00 Without Panic Disorder
		F40.01 With Panic Disorder
	F40.1	Social Phobias
	F40.2	Specific (Isolated) Phobias
	F40.8	Other Phobic Anxiety Disorders
	F40.9	Phobic Anxiety Disorder, Unspecified
F41	**Other Anxiety Disorders**	
	F41.0	Panic Disorder (Episodic Paroxysmal Anxiety)
	F41.1	Generalized Anxiety Disorder
	F41.2	Mixed Anxiety and Depressive Disorder
	F41.3	Other Mixed Anxiety Disorders
	F41.8	Other Specified Anxiety Disorders
	F41.9	Anxiety Disorder, Unspecified

Note. The two categories of anxiety disorders are part of the broader classification of "Neurotic, stress-related, and somatoform disorders." In addition to the two categories of anxiety disorders listed, the broader classification includes disorders such as obsessive-compulsive disorder, reaction to severe stress and adjustment disorders, dissociative disorders, and somatoform disorders.
Source. Adapted from World Health Organization 1992 with permission.

Clinical Features

The typical history of a patient with panic disorder is that of apparently normal functioning until the onset of the first panic attack, which is usually spontaneous. The age of onset is in late adolescence or early adulthood (the 20s). Females predominate over males in a ratio of approximately two to one. The first clinical episode is usually a spontaneous panic attack, spontaneous in that it occurs unexpectedly, without the patient's awareness of a threatening agent in the environment or exposure to a previously known phobic situation (e.g., flying in airplanes, heights, or public speaking). Subsequently, other panic attacks may follow with varying frequency and intensity. Epidemiological evidence indicates that there are moderate numbers of patients, estimated at 9% to 20% of the general population, who experience one or more panic attacks in their lifetimes. The attacks are sometimes described as sporadic, spontaneous, or subclinical. Other persons will experience limited symptom attacks (Klerman et al. 1991).

If a panic attack is of sufficient symptomatic intensity and is accompanied by the cognitive features of dread and foreboding, the patient may seek medical attention in an emergency room, in a general hospital, or from a primary care physician. More than 80% of patients with a diagnosis of panic disorder have consulted a physician within a year of the index episode (Klerman 1990). As more panic attacks occur, the emergence of anticipatory anxiety is typical, with the patient becoming increasingly preoccupied with the fear of another attack and measures that might prevent further attacks. Avoidance behavior frequently develops. Classic agoraphobic situations include using public transportation, driving over bridges or through tunnels, driving on the highway, shopping, and sitting in theaters, churches, and synagogues (hence the term "agoraphobia," literally meaning fear of the marketplace).

According to the views put forth by Klein and embodied in the DSM-III, there is a pathogenetic linkage between recurrent panic attacks and the development of agoraphobia such that the panic attack becomes the aversive conditioning for avoidance behavior in a classic Pavlovian conditioning paradigm. However, as discussed later in this chapter, this linkage between panic attacks and agoraphobia is not universally accepted.

Another clinical feature worthy of note is the high degree of comorbidity of panic disorder with other anxiety disorders, depression, and personality disorders. Comorbidity is discussed later in this chapter.

The long-term clinical course and follow-up of panic disorder are also discussed later.

Clinical Assessment

Assessment

Generally, a thorough history and physical examination are adequate to make the diagnosis of panic disorder in most patients with the disorder. This information is especially true in the typical case of a relatively young patient (age 18 to 45 years) who experiences classic anxiety attacks, avoidance behavior, and often a few depressive symptoms in the context of one or more stressful life events.

Assessment of the patient presenting with panic anxiety will vary according to the professional background of the assessor. If the patient seeks help from a psychiatrist, it is important that there be a careful history of the illness, with family history, social background, and assessment of childhood experiences, such as childhood phobias, degree of behavioral inhibition, and adolescent reactions, including personality type and functioning. Sufficient information about other anxiety disorders must be collected for differential diagnosis and assessment of comorbidity. It is recommended that a physical examination and laboratory screen be done and a medical history obtained. In most patients, a few laboratory tests, such as a complete blood count, blood chemistry panel, and thyroid function tests, are adequate.

On the other hand, a person with panic symptoms often presents to a primary care physician or a nonpsychiatric medical specialist. In that event, after the appropriate medical evaluations have been completed, the patient usually should be referred to a psychiatrist for confirmation of the diagnosis and recommendations for treatment. (See Table 6 for recommended evaluations.)

At times, the focus of a patient on a specific complaint, such as chest pain, dizziness, or epigastric pain, will necessitate further testing (e.g., an upper gastrointestinal [GI] series or electrocardiogram [ECG]). If the patient presents at the emergency room of a general hospital with severe symptoms suggestive of possible heart disease, the medical examination, at a minimum, should include a physical examination, ECG, serum enzymes, and blood count. Other presentations may suggest asthma, epilepsy, or irritable bowel syndrome and should be investigated accordingly. Negative results of medical tests can reassure the clinician and patient that other medical disorders are not present. On the other hand, conducting a large number of tests can be costly and may further reinforce patient hypochondriasis.

Differential Diagnosis

Other psychiatric and medical disorders can be confused with panic disorder. Because panic disorder is diagnosed on the basis of descriptive criteria rather than a laboratory test, these other disorders need to be ruled out before the diagnosis of panic disorder can be made. The most important of those disorders are discussed next.

Psychiatric Disorders

Differentiation of panic disorder from other psychiatric disorders, particularly depression, is often difficult. Other psychiatric disorders that sometimes mimic panic disorder are listed in Table 7 and discussed in the following paragraphs.

Depression. Patients with primary depression often experience agitation, signs of anxiety, and panic attacks. To complicate clinical as-

---

Table 6. Assessment of patient presenting with panic anxiety

Psychiatric assessment
- Family history
- Developmental history
    Childhood phobia
    Behavioral inhibitions
    Premorbid personality
- Suicidal ideation, attempts
- Comorbidity
    Other anxiety disorder
    Depression
    Alcoholism
    Drug abuse

Mental status exam

Medical assessment
- Medical history
- Physical examination
- Laboratory tests
    Electrocardiogram
    Serum cardiac enzyme
    Complete blood count
    Electroencephalogram
    Thyroid status

Current social functioning and quality of life

sessment, patients with panic disorder sometimes acquire depression secondarily. However, there are several clinical differences between the two disorders: 1) Patients with panic disorder do not usually have the full range of vegetative symptoms that depressive patients have (e.g., they may have difficulty falling asleep but usually do not experience early morning awakening); 2) diurnal mood fluctuation is uncommon in anxiety disorders; and 3) purely anxious patients do not lose the capacity to enjoy life or to be cheered up.

Atypical depression is characterized by a lack of endogenous features, which makes its differentiation from panic disorder difficult. Patients with atypical depression can be easily cheered up, but their mood tends to worsen faster than that of patients with panic disorder. Panic disorder and atypical depression may coexist.

Depersonalization disorder.   Patients with depersonalization disorder have episodes of depersonalization-derealization, but they do not have the other symptoms of a panic attack.

Medical Disorders

As shown in Table 7, a differential diagnosis may have to be made between panic attacks and several medical conditions. The most important of those medical conditions include thyroid disease, mitral valve prolapse (MVP), illicit drug use, caffeinism, and side effects of prescription medications (Katon and Roy-Byrne 1989). In recent controlled studies, no evidence of abnormally increased thyroid hormone levels was found in patients with panic disorder. However, persons with hyperthyroidism often experience anxiety, tachycardia, palpita-

Table 7.   Differential diagnosis of panic attacks

Psychiatric	Medical
◆ Adjustment disorder with anxious mood	◆ Coronary artery disease
	◆ Epilepsy
◆ Generalized anxiety	◆ Irritable bowel
◆ Simple phobia (heights, flying, elevators, closed spaces, etc.)	◆ Mitral valve prolapse
	◆ Thyroid
	◆ Drug use or side effects
◆ Social phobia	
◆ Public-speaking phobia	

tions, sweating, dyspnea, irritability, diarrhea, and diffuse anxiety.

Panic disorder is associated with an increased prevalence of MVP. However, in the vast majority of cases, MVP is mild, is not associated with thickened mitral valve leaflets, and is principally an echocardiographic finding (Katon 1989). This mild type of MVP has little clinical relevance and does not require prophylactic antibiotic treatment, except in rare cases in which mitral valve thickness is increased to 5 mm or more. This thickness may be caused by increased heart rate, catecholamine excretion, and increased adrenergic tone.

Panic disorder frequently is unrecognized in patients with comorbid panic disorder and MVP. Many of these patients are prescribed beta-adrenergic blocking agents for the MVP, which may have a mild anxiolytic effect but may precipitate or worsen depressive symptoms. A change to more specific treatment for panic disorder usually leads to rapid amelioration of panic attacks and cardiorespiratory symptoms.

In some persons, a first anxiety attack may be precipitated by the use of marijuana, cocaine, amphetamines, or hallucinogens. The frightening somatic or cognitive symptoms that can occur with use of these drugs may provoke an anxiety response to the perceived loss of control. Alternatively, some of the physiological effects of these agents may stimulate specific brain receptors associated with anxiety. For example, cocaine can cause the acute release of serotonin, norepinephrine, and dopamine and block their reuptake (Katon and Roy-Byrne 1989). Chronic cocaine use depletes these catecholamines. Several researchers hypothesized that chronic cocaine-induced depletion of biogenic amines could alter the equilibrium of the noradrenergic system by reducing the activity of inhibitory inputs (Aronson and Craig 1986). This reduced inhibitory input can increase the susceptibility of the chronic cocaine user to panic attacks. Marijuana causes a well-documented increase in heart rate, probably by beta-adrenergic cardiovascular stimulation (Beaconsfield et al. 1972). This side effect may precipitate severe anxiety in susceptible users. Finally, withdrawal from sedative-hypnotics, alcohol, or opiates can cause symptoms that are difficult to distinguish from anxiety attacks. People with panic disorder are more susceptible to the anxiogenic effects of caffeine. Several studies showed that subjects with panic disorder tend to decrease their use of caffeine, and case reports also suggested that hypercaffeinism can precipitate anxiety disorders and panic attacks that are often reversible when caffeine intake is decreased (Greden 1974).

Interface With General Medicine

Help-Seeking and Somatization

Although panic disorder is now considered to be a psychiatric condition, most persons with panic disorder are not seen by psychiatrists or other mental health professionals but, rather, are seen in the general health sector by nonpsychiatric medical specialists (cardiologists, neurologists, or gastroenterologists) and primary care physicians.

Moreover, panic disorder can be confused with other disorders (see Differential Diagnosis) or can be comorbid with other disorders (see later discussions in this chapter).

Data from the Epidemiologic Catchment Area (ECA) have shown that respondents in the community with panic disorder are frequent users of medical services (Klerman 1991). Over a 1-year period, 86% of persons with panic disorder and 67% of persons with panic attacks, compared with 31% of persons with other psychiatric disorders, sought treatment from health care professionals. In addition, patients with panic disorder, when compared with patients with any other psychiatric disorder, had highest use of general medical services for specialty mental health services over the previous 6 months.

Studies of patients selected for their frequent use of medical services also found robust prevalence rates of panic disorder. In a recent study of 767 frequent users (patients among the highest 10% of users of ambulatory care) at two large primary care health maintenance organization clinics, 50% of those patients were found to have significant psychological distress (Katon et al. 1990). This group of frequent users of medical care was responsible for 29% of outpatient primary care visits, 52% of outpatient specialty visits, 25% of all prescriptions, and 48% of all inpatient hospital days over a 1-year period. The Diagnostic Interview Schedule (L. N. Robins et al. 1981) was administered to assess 119 of these distressed patients: 12% met the DSM-III-R criteria for current panic disorder, and 30% met criteria for lifetime panic disorder.

Persons with panic attacks have also been found to be overrepresented among primary care patients, with a prevalence of 6% to 8% in several studies in which the Diagnostic Interview Schedule or other structured psychiatric interviews were used (Katon et al. 1992). However, these patients usually do not undergo diagnosis or treatment for panic. In response to the lack of accurate diagnosis and treatment of patients with panic disorder, the National Institute of Mental Health (in the United States) has launched a national campaign entitled "The Panic Disorder Prevention and Public Education Program" to try to better educate primary care physicians and the public about the currently available effective treatments for this distressing disorder.

Misdiagnosis and Undertreatment

Many patients with panic disorder who present to medical practitioners with symptoms such as chest pain and irritable bowel syndrome undergo costly and often invasive medical testing before the correct diagnosis is made. For instance, 10% to 30% of patients who undergo angiograms in the United States have a negative workup. Several studies have determined that approximately one-third to one-half of patients with chest pain and negative angiograms have panic disorder. Angiograms cost approximately $3,000 in the United States, and approximately 1 million angiograms are performed there yearly. If, conservatively, 10% of those angiograms are negative and one-third of the patients with negative angiograms have panic disorder, the cost of testing panic disorder patients who present with chest pain would be more than $90 million per year. Moreover, two studies demonstrated that patients with chest pain who had negative cardiac work-ups and panic disorder but who were still experiencing cardiac symptoms 2 years later were significantly more likely to report vocational and social impairment than those who did not have panic disorder (Beitman et al. 1991).

Persons with irritable bowel syndrome represent approximately one-quarter to one-half of all patients examined by gastroenterologists. These patients frequently undergo upper and lower GI series and endoscopy. Better recognition and more appropriate treatment of panic disorder could result in a large cost savings for these patients. Pharmacological studies of panic disorder have consistently documented extremely high pretreatment scores on psychological measures of somatization in patients with panic disorder and, after effective treatment, a reduction in their scores to normal levels (Fava et al. 1988; Noyes et al. 1986a). In patients with irritable bowel syndrome, pharmacological and cognitive-behavioral treatments targeted at psychological distress have been shown effective and hold promise for the future (Creed and Guthrie 1989).

Panic disorder can also be present concurrently with chronic medical illness, such as diabetes mellitus, coronary artery disease, or asthma. The autonomic arousal associated with panic disorder may lead to significant worsening of a formerly well-controlled chronic medical illness and a subsequent increase in medical utilization (Katon and Roy-Byrne 1989). For example, Dirks and colleagues (1980) found that patients with asthma and severe anxiety have three times as many hospitalizations as asthmatic patients with similar degrees of physiological asthma but low levels of anxiety.

Recent studies of patients with irritable bowel syndrome (Fossey and Lydiard 1990; Walker et al. 1990), negative angiograms after chest pain (Beitman et al. 1987; Katon et al. 1988), medically unexplained dizziness, migraine headache (Merikangas et al. 1990; Stewart et al. 1989), and chronic fatigue syndrome (Katon 1991; Manu et al. 1991) have all shown high rates of panic disorder in those patient populations.

In the ECA study, respondents in the community with either panic disorder or infrequent panic attacks were found to be more frequent users of emergency medical services and were more likely to be hospitalized for physical problems than persons not experiencing panic attacks (Klerman 1991). Patients with panic disorder often attribute their autonomic symptoms to cardiac disease (e.g., a heart attack) or a neurological illness (e.g., a cerebrovascular accident) and therefore visit emergency services. A recent study of 100 patients who had visited emergency services for a medically unexplained somatic complaint demonstrated a prevalence of panic disorder and generalized anxiety disorder sixfold higher than an emergency room control group (Klein et al. 1992, in press). Studies by Wulsin and colleagues (1988) of patients in the emergency room with chest pain who had negative medical workups also showed an extremely high prevalence of panic disorder.

In addition to somatization and frequent medical utilization, delays in the diagnosis of panic disorder can frequently lead to the development of associated comorbid psychiatric conditions, an increased likelihood of suicide attempts, impaired social and marital functioning, increased use of psychoactive medications, and financial dependence (Markowitz et al. 1989). Patients with panic disorder have an increased risk of suicide attempts compared with patients with other psychiatric disorders (Weissman et al. 1989). Panic disorder is also associated with a decline in some social activities, such as time spent on hobbies. In the ECA study, patients with panic disorder had an increased risk of financial dependence (Markowitz et al. 1989).

Panic disorder is also associated with an increased risk of comorbid psychiatric conditions, which in many cases develop secondary to panic attacks. In the ECA study, approximately one-third of patients with panic disorder had an associated major depression, one-third had agoraphobia, one-quarter abused alcohol, and one-sixth abused drugs (Klerman 1991). The presence of a comorbid psychiatric disorder is associated with increased social and occupational dysfunction and a poorer response to psychopharmacological treatment.

Epidemiology and Familial Risk

There is now considerable information on the epidemiology and familial risk of panic disorder drawn from large probability samples from the community, both in the United States and cross-nationally, and from family studies undertaken independently at several centers.

Rates (Prevalence)

Information on the epidemiology of panic disorder in the United States comes from the ECA study (Robins and Regier 1991), a community survey conducted in the early 1980s of more than 18,000 adults, ages 18 years and older, living in five cities (New Haven, Connecticut; Baltimore, Maryland; St. Louis, Missouri; Durham, North Carolina; and Los Angeles, California). Although the study was conducted independently at each site, similar methodology and identical diagnostic procedures were used at all sites.

The study showed that, over a lifetime, about one-fourth of the subjects believed that they were nervous people; 9.3% had isolated panic attacks; 3.6% had experienced panic attacks not meeting the full criteria for panic disorder because of insufficient symptoms, duration, or frequency of attacks; and about 1.5% met the DSM-III criteria for panic disorder at some time in their life. About one-third of the subjects with panic attacks also met the criteria for agoraphobia. This proportion was consistent by sex. These rates are remarkably consistent with the rates found in other epidemiological studies, conducted with similar diagnostic methods in Germany; Puerto Rico; France; Edmonton, Canada; New Zealand; and Seoul, Korea (Canino et al. 1987;

Faravelli et al. 1989; Joyce et al. 1989; Lee et al. 1987; Weissman et al. 1989; Wittchen 1986b). The rates were lower in Taiwan (Hwu et al. 1989). However, the rates of most mental disorders, for reasons that are unclear, were lower in Taiwan.

Many persons—about 3% to 4% of adults—have recurrent panic attacks that do not meet the DSM-III criteria for panic disorder (Klerman et al. 1991). Approximately 10% of adults have isolated panic attacks. There seems to be a gradient for the degree of disability and help-seeking behavior that correlates roughly to the number and intensity of attacks.

Risk Factors

Several risk factors for panic attacks and panic disorder have been identified.

1. *Sex.* There is predominance of females over males who have panic disorder.
2. *Age at onset.* Panic disorder is a disorder of young adults, with the first panic attack occurring most often in late adolescence to early adulthood (the third decade) and panic disorder occurring in the mid to late 20s. There are a growing number of reports that panic disorder can occur in prepubertal children, although it is uncommon in that group (Ballenger et al. 1988; Moreau and Weissman 1992; Moreau et al. 1989). There appears to be a decrease in onset with later age, with first onset infrequent after the age of 45 years.
3. *Medical illness.* As is discussed next, certain medical conditions including epilepsy, stroke, thyroid disease, and MVP are associated with an increased risk of panic disorder.

Family History as a Risk Factor

A review of family studies, using specified diagnostic criteria, shows the highly familial nature of panic disorder and suggests evidence for a genetic cause. The population-based lifetime rates of panic disorder cross-nationally range between 1.2 in 100 and 2 in 100, whereas the lifetime rates of panic disorder in the first-degree relatives of patients with panic disorder range between 7 in 100 and 20 in 100 (Crowe et al. 1983; E. L. Harris et al. 1983; Hopper et al. 1987; W. Maier, personal communication, April 1990; Moran and Andrews 1985; Noyes et al.

1986b; Torgersen 1983; Weissman 1990). Absolute rates of panic disorder vary according to the strictness of the diagnostic criteria used. In all cases, rates of panic disorder are significantly higher in the relatives of patients with panic disorder compared with the relatives of control subjects.

A twin study published by Torgersen, although based on small samples, suggested a higher rate of panic disorder in the monozygotic co-twins of panic probands than in the dizygotic twins. A similar association was not seen for anxiety disorder without panic disorder. A considerably larger twin study using clinical diagnosis in a female sample is currently being conducted by Kendler; preliminary results that give more evidence for genetic cause are reported in Chapter 3. The full results of the study are not yet available.

Evidence from family and twin studies supports the separation of panic disorder and generalized anxiety disorder (Crowe et al. 1988; E. L. Harris et al. 1983; Noyes et al. 1986b; Torgersen 1983), as is discussed in Chapters 3 and 4. Evidence for a relation between panic disorder and major depression is still unclear, as is the mode of transmission of panic disorder.

The high lifetime prevalence of panic disorder, the strong evidence for vertical transmission, and the identification of potential biological markers have increased interest in the application of modern genetic linkage techniques to the study of the disorder. Several genetic linkage studies of panic disorder are ongoing, but no results are yet available. (For a discussion of the genetic theories of the origin of panic, see Chapter 3).

Cross-National and Cross-Cultural Considerations

The initial descriptions of what today is considered a panic attack were made in the United Kingdom and North America, leading many observers to question the universality of the condition. This discussion revived the 19th-century concept of neurasthenia as a "disease of American civilization." Many European and South American psychiatrists reported that panic disorder did not occur in their countries.

However, several culture-specific syndromes, such as *kuru* in Malaysia and Indonesia and *kajak-angst* among Eskimos, have been discussed as cultural variants of panic disorder. Fright disorders such as *susto* in Latin America and *latah* in Southeast Asia may be panic attacks; further investigations are called for (Katschnig and Amering 1990). With widening use in the mid-1980s of DSM-III criteria in many countries other than the United States and, in particular, with the experience of the Cross-National Collaborative Panic Study (CNCPS), it is now established that there are patients with panic attacks and panic disorder in all societies that have been studied (Katschnig 1991). Moreover, as noted previously, recent epidemiological studies in New Zealand, Germany, Puerto Rico, Canada, Korea, and other countries that have used DSM-III or DSM-III-R criteria demonstrated similar prevalence rates (Weissman 1991; Wittchen 1986a), with no major differences in risk factors or age at onset.

Uncomplicated and Comorbid Panic Disorder

The concept of comorbidity originated in general medical epidemiology, particularly in the work of Feinstein (1970), who observed that the outcome of a clinical trial often varied with the presence of another diagnosis in addition to the condition under study. Since the development of the DSM-III-R, the concept has gained prominence in the psychiatric literature, where increasing attention has been paid to comorbidity in clinical, epidemiological, and family studies. The DSM-III-R suspended many of the diagnostic hierarchies of the DSM-II, DSM-III, and ICD (Maser and Cloninger 1984). For example, if panic attacks developed during an episode of depressive illness, the earlier diagnostic systems considered them part of the depression rather than a separate disorder. However, when the hierarchies were suspended by the DSM-III-R, both disorders could be diagnosed. It then became apparent that, for many disorders, particularly the anxiety and mood disorders, pure or uncomplicated cases were relatively uncommon and high degrees of comorbidity existed.

Uncomplicated Panic Disorder

Panic disorder meeting full DSM-III, DSM-III-R, or ICD criteria but not accompanied by any comorbid condition (uncomplicated panic disorder) appears to be relatively uncommon. In the ECA study, about 25% of the patients with panic disorder meeting DSM-III criteria did not have a comorbid condition. However, panic attacks that fall short of specific diagnostic criteria for frequency of occurrence or number of symptoms appear to be quite common (Klerman et al. 1990). There is not yet a consensus whether these "subsyndromal" cases represent the mild end of the panic disorder spectrum or are a different or merely normal phenomenon.

Comorbidity With Agoraphobia

Agoraphobia is traditionally defined as fear and avoidance of a cluster of situations that vary from patient to patient but in which there are clearly identifiable recurrent themes. From a review of factor-analytic studies, Marks and colleagues (1989) concluded that the core of the cluster consists of public places, such as streets, stores, public transportation vehicles, auditoriums, and crowded areas. At the periphery of the cluster are situations such as being in elevators, in tunnels, on bridges, in open spaces, and at heights. Being alone or going into such situations alone is especially difficult for persons with agoraphobia. In severe forms of agoraphobia, the disorder can be completely incapacitating, with the patient unable to work and limited in social and family activities. In its most extreme form, agoraphobia confines patients to the home, as in the image of the housebound homemaker.

Investigators agree that the frequency of comorbidity of agoraphobia and panic attacks is high, but the relation between the two disorders is debated. As mentioned previously, in the "American view," spontaneous panic attacks are the core and initiating event of panic disorder. Secondary anticipatory anxiety and phobic avoidance develop frequently but not in all patients. In the "European view," as expressed by writers such as Marks and colleagues (1989) and Roth and Argyle (1988), phobic attitudes are the core of the disorder and frequently but not necessarily progress to panic disorder. In the "American view," the sequence of events should always be panic attacks first and anticipatory anxiety and phobias later if at all, whereas according to the "European view" symptoms can develop in any order.

The empirical evidence that panic attacks usually precede agoraphobia is strong. However, it has not been firmly established that this sequence always occurs or, conversely, that no phobia from the agoraphobia cluster ever precedes the onset of panic disorder. A study by Marks's group (Lelliott et al. 1989) found that phobic avoidance preceded panic attacks in only 23% of cases. It is not known whether one or more specific phobias from the agoraphobia cluster may be a risk factor predicting a later onset of panic disorder. Investigators who fol-

low the DSM-III-R system would probably presume that any circum-
scribed phobias, even of situations from the "agoraphobia cluster,"
that begin before the onset of panic attacks were not part of agoraphobia but rather a separate simple phobia.

Agoraphobia without panic attacks should be rare or nonexistent
according to the "American view" but not uncommon according to the
"European view." There is general agreement that agoraphobia without a history of panic disorder is uncommon in clinical samples,
whereas epidemiology surveys suggest a high prevalence in the general population. However, the latter finding may reflect the sampling
and selection processes used. Studies by Himle and co-workers (1989)
found that DSM-III-R simple phobias of the type that also belong to
the "agoraphobic cluster" are associated with mean ages at onset more
similar to those associated with agoraphobia than with other simple
phobias. Furthermore, they frequently begin with what would otherwise be described as a spontaneous panic attack occurring while the
person is in the situation of which he or she then becomes phobic. The
difference between those simple phobias and panic disorder with agoraphobia is that the person does not have panic attacks in other situations and does not acquire an extensive network of phobias. On the
basis of these and other data, it has been proposed that at least some
simple phobias of this type may actually be mild cases of panic disorder with agoraphobia.

In studies on pharmacological treatment of panic disorder, it does
not appear that the presence of agoraphobia limits the response to
medication prescribed for panic attacks. Most medications that block
panic attacks also ameliorate avoidance behavior, help-seeking behavior, and phobic avoidance.

Comorbidity With Other Anxiety Disorders

Massion and colleagues (in press) looked at rates of past and current
alcohol or substance abuse in a sample of 357 subjects with panic disorder with or without agoraphobia, or general anxiety disorder, or
both. Of the subjects without general anxiety disorder, 44% of those
with panic disorder without agoraphobia reported a history of alcohol
or substance abuse, compared to 27% of those with panic disorder with
agoraphobia. Those with both panic disorder and general anxiety disorder (with or without agoraphobia) had an even lower rate of 22%.
The finding of a higher rate for panic disorder without agoraphobia

compared to panic disorder with agoraphobia is contradictory to the findings of Kushner and colleagues (1990) and Himle and Hill (1991).

Aside from agoraphobia, the anxiety symptoms most commonly reported in association with panic disorder are symptoms resembling generalized anxiety disorder (Aronson and Logue 1987; Brier et al. 1986; Fava et al. 1988; Lelliott et al. 1989; Marks 1987; Uhde et al. 1985) and social phobia (Kendler et al. 1992b).

Social phobia is associated with an earlier age at onset (mean of about 15 years) and usually precedes the development of panic disorder or agoraphobia (Schneier et al. 1992). Generalized anxiety disorder (GAD)-like symptoms, however, can either precede or follow panic disorder. Obsessive-compulsive disorder or posttraumatic stress disorder also can occur concurrently with panic disorder, but these comorbidities have not been extensively studied.

Comorbidity With Depression

Two major lines of evidence suggest a close connection between panic disorder and depressive disorders. The first is that many investigators have noted high rates of comorbidity of the two disorders, both concurrently and on a life history basis (Brier et al. 1984, 1985, 1986; Grunhaus et al. 1988; Robins and Regier 1991; Roth and Argyle 1988; Stavrakaki and Vargo 1986; Wittchen et al. 1992). Either disorder can occur first, or both can occur simultaneously. However, more commonly, it is thought that panic disorder occurs first and is followed by depressive episodes several years later.

The second line of evidence, as noted elsewhere in this review, is that most drugs that are effective for treating depression (TCAs, MAOIs, and selective serotonin reuptake blockers) are also effective for treating panic disorder. Two exceptions, on the basis of single published studies, appear to be buspirone (Sheehan et al. 1990) and trazodone. The converse, however, is not true. High-potency benzodiazepines are very effective for treating panic disorder; however, although they have been reported to have some efficacy for treating depression, they are not, on the whole, very good antidepressants.

Biological marker studies have shown that psychophysiological responses to panic disorder and depression are sometimes similar and sometimes different. A blunted growth hormone response to a test dose of clonidine is about equally characteristic of panic disorder and major depression. On the other hand, hypercortisolemia and shortened REM latency are very characteristic of major depression but much less so of panic disorder.

Comorbidity With Personality Disorders

The clinical studies of personality and anxiety have been thoroughly reviewed by Roy-Byrne and colleagues (1988) and Mavissakalian and Jones (1990). Personality disorders are more common in psychiatric patients than in general practice patients and appear to determine treatment-seeking behavior. Some studies of panic disorder patients do not clearly distinguish their personality traits from the personality traits of other psychiatric patients or healthy control subjects (Mavissakalian and Jones 1990; Sciuto et al. 1991). In fact, one study provided evidence for preserving the concept of a general neurotic syndrome (Tyrer et al. 1983).

Other studies indicate that patients with panic disorder-agoraphobia are overanxious, avoidant, dependent, and unassertive and lack self-confidence. Certain personality measures, specifically emotional strength, interpersonal dependence, and social self-confidence, may reportedly improve as panic scores improve. Intolerance of being alone, hypersensitivity, and passive resistance can also improve with treatment. It also appears that panic disorder with agoraphobia is more likely to be accompanied by personality disorders than panic disorder uncomplicated by agoraphobic avoidance (Noyes et al. 1990; Reich et al. 1987; Starcevic 1991).

Comorbidity With Alcoholism

Kushner and associates (1990) performed a meta-analysis of several studies of clinical samples and found median rates of alcoholism of 20.2% among patients with agoraphobia and 7.6% among patients with panic disorder compared with a rate of alcoholism of 13.3% in the general population found in the ECA study. In reanalyzing data from the ECA study, Himle and Hill (1991) found an alcoholism rate of 31.5% among subjects with agoraphobia and panic attacks meeting DSM-III criteria and 20.4% among patients with panic disorder but no agoraphobia.

Massion and colleagues (in press) reported on 294 subjects with panic disorder with and without agoraphobia from the Harvard Anxiety Research Program (HARP), a prospective, naturalistic longitudinal study of anxiety disorders. Forty-three percent of the study group had another anxiety disorder at intake; 54% had either another anxiety disorder or major depression.

The apparent association between panic disorder and alcoholism may be inflated because of the occurrence of anxiety and panic attacks as a result of alcohol withdrawal. In an effort to correct for this possibility, some investigators suggest that only those cases in which panic disorder or agoraphobia had been present during a period of abstinence from alcohol of at least 3 months are diagnosed. By that criterion, they found no cases of panic disorder or agoraphobia among 191 alcoholic male veterans. In a study of an exclusively female alcoholic population, Nunes and co-workers (1988) included only those cases with active symptoms during prolonged abstinence from alcohol. They found that 32% had panic disorder with agoraphobia, whereas 8% had panic disorder without agoraphobia. When only those cases with an onset of alcoholism subsequent to that of panic disorder with agoraphobia were included, the association between alcoholism and panic disorder-agoraphobia was still higher than expected from the prevalence of each disorder in the general population.

Rates of association should be determined separately for each sex because panic disorder and agoraphobia occur more frequently in women, and alcoholism occurs more frequently in men. The risk of alcoholism appears to be consistently higher in agoraphobia than in uncomplicated panic disorder, and persons with agoraphobia may represent a very high percentage of women with alcoholism.

Comorbidity With Medical Conditions

Panic disorder can be present concurrently with any of a number of medical conditions, as has already been discussed. Additionally, it appears that the presence of one disorder can increase the risk that the other disorder will occur. For example, there is evidence that the prevalence of panic disorder is higher in patients with cardiac symptoms, thyroid disease, migraine headache, or irritable bowel syndrome than in the general population. Panic disorder is also more prevalent in patients with MVP, although asymptomatic patients with MVP had no higher risk of panic disorder than control subjects (Katon and Roy-Byrne 1989).

The converse notion that the prevalence of medical disorders in patients with panic disorder is higher than that in the general population has been studied extensively. Wells and associates (1989) analyzed data on 2,552 persons from the Los Angeles site of the ECA study to determine whether chronic medical illnesses would be more prevalent in persons with depressive and anxiety disorders meeting DSM-III criteria than in those without psychiatric illness. The analysis compared 841 persons who had one or more chronic medical conditions with 1,711 persons who had no medical condition.

Estimates were provided of the prevalence of eight chronic medical conditions in persons with any of three categories of psychiatric disorders (anxiety, affective disorders, and substance abuse) and in persons without any psychiatric disorder. The chronic medical conditions were chronic lung disease, diabetes mellitus, heart disease, hypertension, arthritis, physical handicap, cancer, and stroke.

Wells and associates (1989) found that persons with a lifetime psychiatric disorder (affective disorder, anxiety, or substance abuse) had a significantly higher lifetime prevalence of chronic medical conditions compared with persons with no lifetime psychiatric disorder. Results also showed that persons with recent anxiety disorders had a greater prevalence of any current chronic medical condition. This finding suggests that persons with recent anxiety disorders should be carefully evaluated for diabetes, heart disease, and arthritis. Weissman and associates (1990) examined the New Haven, Connecticut, data from the ECA study to determine whether the risk of stroke was higher for panic disorder patients than for other persons. Of the New Haven subjects, 60 had lifetime panic disorder; 1,036 had some other psychiatric disorder; and 3,778 had no psychiatric disorder. The risk for stroke in persons with a diagnosis of panic disorder was more than twice that in persons with some other psychiatric disorder or no psychiatric disorder. These findings were consistent with clinical studies showing an association between panic disorder and cardiovascular or cerebrovascular events (Weissman et al. 1990).

Clinical Course and Follow-Up

Panic disorder is considered by the general public and by many clinicians to be a short-lived disorder. However, the results of a number of carefully conducted medium- and long-term follow-up studies belie this notion. In fact, panic disorder is often a chronic disorder associated with significant psychosocial disabilities. If panic disorder is not treated, it seems to follow a variable course (spontaneous periods of exacerbation followed by spontaneous periods, on the order of months to years, of improvement). Currently, there is no reliable predictor of those patients in whom agoraphobia will develop.

Short-term treatment (e.g., up to 12 weeks), with the psychological or pharmacological methods described in Chapter 5, effectively blocks panic attacks in 70% to 90% of patients but is associated with relatively high rates (e.g., 20% to 80%) of relapse. Some clinicians (e.g., Ballenger 1990), however, proposed that the short-term treatment model is inappropriate; rather, treatment, like the course of the disease itself, should be viewed as long term (6 to 12 months or more) from the outset.

Information is available on the long-term course of panic disorder, both before widespread use of current psychological and pharmacological treatments and after such treatments were introduced. The results of five longitudinal studies completed between 1938 and 1957 (Blair et al. 1957; Eitinger 1955; A. Harris 1938; Miles et al. 1951; Wheeler et al. 1950) showed that rates of recovery were approximately one-third at the follow-up assessment. The average follow-up period was approximately 10 years. A large number of patients, however, continued to have substantial symptomatology and disability many years after initial evaluation and treatment. Poorest long-term outcome was usually associated with severest symptomatology and debilitation at index.

In several studies (Buller et al. 1986; Coryell et al. 1991; Katschnig et al. 1991; Krieg et al. 1987; Maier and Buller 1988; Mavissakalian and Michelson 1986b; Nagy et al. 1989; Noyes et al. 1989a, 1990), approximately 40% of patients were fully recovered or markedly improved at follow-up assessment. The average follow-up period in these studies was approximately 3.5 years. Approximately one in five patients was severely debilitated at follow-up. For example, in the study reported by Katschnig (which was a follow-up of 367 patients over a 2- to 6-year period after entering the CNCPS), only about one-fifth of patients had a severe, chronic course (18.6%), whereas 31% had recovered and stayed well; the remainder followed an intermediate course (Katschnig et al. 1991). As was the case with the earlier studies, the most severely impaired patients at follow-up were those that were most severely impaired at index.

When studies from the premodern and current treatment eras were compared in a meta-analysis (Hirschfeld 1992), the number of very poor outcomes appeared to decrease in the later studies (see Tables 8 and 9), suggesting the possibility that the most severely ill patients responded to the new treatments. However, rates of full recovery did not change. Reasons proposed for the lack of change in full recovery are that 1) the newer treatments are effective over the short term but not the long term; and 2) the newer treatments were not continued for a sufficient period of time. The concept of continuing treatment to extend recovery has been borne out in depression. In view of other parallels between panic disorder and depression, the concept may be applicable to panic disorder as well.

A recent study, the Harvard/Brown Anxiety Research Program, observed, for a 3-year period, more than 700 patients who presented for treatment at 1 of 11 sites in the United States (Keller 1992, submitted for publication). The study data analyzed thus far indicate that patients with panic disorder have high levels of chronicity, relapse, and comorbidity with other anxiety disorders and with depression. Moreover, the presence of comorbid depression was predictive of severe psychopathology and considerable psychosocial impairment, as reflected in measures of occupational, home, and leisure functioning.

Table 8. Premodern treatment era studies (total N = 367)

Study	Diagnosis	N	Years of follow-up	Outcome % (n) Well or markedly improved	Moderate symptoms	Poor
Harris 1938[a]	Various AS	123	10–12	31 (38)	9 (11)	47 (58)
Wheeler et al. 1950	NA	60	20+	12 (7)	73 (44)	15 (9)
Miles et al. 1951	AN	62	2–12	23 (14)	36 (22)	42 (26)
Eitinger 1955	AN	29	10+	41 (12)	34 (10)	24 (7)
Blair et al. 1957[b]	AS	93	1–6	52 (48)	28 (26)	8 (7)
Total		367		32 (119)	31 (113)	29 (107)

[a] 13% of these subjects were deceased at follow-up.
[b] 12% of these subjects were deceased or not traceable at follow-up.
AS = anxiety states; NA = neurocirculatory asthenia; AN = anxiety neurosis.
Source. Adapted from Hirschfeld 1992, pp. 105–119, with permission.

Table 9. Modern treatment era studies

Study	Diagnosis	N	Years of follow-up	Outcome % (n)		
				Well or markedly improved	Moderate symptoms	Poor
Katschnig et al. 1991	PD, AG	220	2–6	31 (68)	50 (110)	19 (42)
Noyes et al. 1990; Coryell et al. 1991	PD	89	3	47 (41)	49 (44)	6 (5)
Nagy et al. 1989	PD, AG	60	1.5–4	43 (26)	38 (23)	18 (11)
Noyes et al. 1989a	PD, AG	107	1–4	62 (66)	28 (30)	10 (11)
Maier and Buller 1988[a]; Buller et al. 1986[a]	PD, AG	77	1	43 (33)		
Krieg et al. 1987	AN	40	6–8	5 (2)	28 (11)	68 (27)
Mavissakalian and Michelson 1986b[a]	PD, AG	41	2	59 (24)		
Total		634		41 (260) (N = 634)	42[b] (218) (N = 516)	19 (96) (N = 516)

Note. PD = panic disorder; AG = agoraphobia; AN = anxiety neurosis.
[a] The number of subjects with moderate and poor symptoms was not reported in this study.
[b] Excludes Buller et al. 1986; Maier and Buller 1988; and Mavissakalian and Michelson 1986.
Source. Adapted from Hirschfeld 1992, pp. 105–119, with permission.

Medical Morbidity and Mortality

Although patients with panic attacks seek medical help because of their fears of immediate death, this fear is unfounded in almost all instances, and the patient is judged by medical authorities not to be in any immediate danger. However, epidemiological self-report data suggest a possible increase in cerebrovascular episodes in such patients as well as possible arrhythmias and cardiovascular disease. Studies also suggest that panic disorder may lead to physiological worsening of cardiac illness, with more frequent episodes of chest pain (Katon 1990). The most remarkable finding reported in one study was that 83% of a sample of 35 patients with cardiomyopathy met DSM-III criteria for panic disorder compared with 16% of the control group awaiting a new heart because of postinfarction heart failure (Cassem 1990).

A study that examined the effect of panic disorder on other medical illnesses showed that panic disorder either worsened the medical illness or was associated with continued physiological symptoms that mimicked the medical illness after the illness improved. In either case, panic disorder was shown to cause an increase in the use of medical services that often included costly testing as well as additional distress (Katon and Roy-Byrne 1989).

Several studies determined that there is a significant increase in deaths from unnatural causes, particularly suicide, and that there is also an increased risk of cardiovascular disease as well as respiratory disorders in persons afflicted with panic disorder (Coryell et al. 1986; Kerr et al. 1969; Martin et al. 1985; Zandbergen et al. 1991). Panic disorder is also associated with increases in GI symptoms and irritable bowel symptoms (Noyes et al. 1990). Panic disorder affects many aspects of a patient's general health and because overall health is the greatest predictor of mortality, it is reasonable to conclude that mortality rates are increased by panic disorder.

Coryell and associates conducted a study of 155 outpatients who sought treatment at the University of Iowa Hospitals and Clinics between 1968 and 1972 and who were given a diagnosis of anxiety disorder (Coryell et al. 1986). This study was an attempt to replicate their earlier 35-year follow-up of inpatients; in this study they found that the mortality rate among men with panic disorder was greater than that expected on the basis of population statistics. Patients with any physical illness that could cause anxiety symptoms were not included in the anxiety disorder group or control group.

The mortality follow-up was performed 12 years after the original clinical contact with the original patients; 81.3% of the anxiety group and 85.4% of the control group were located and mortality status was determined. Death certificates were obtained for those subjects who had died during follow-up. Each death certificate was assigned to one of five categories according to the cause of death: unnatural causes (including suicide), circulatory system disease, neoplastic disease, infectious disease, or other natural causes. Mortality rates between study groups and the Iowa population were then compared. All deaths among men with anxiety disorders were due to cardiovascular disease or suicide; all deaths among men from the control group were due to other causes. Factors such as MVP and alcohol abuse, when they were investigated, were not considered as likely reasons for the excess cardiovascular mortality. The results suggest, as did the results of their first study, that men with panic disorder are at an increased risk for death from suicide and for cardiovascular disease.

Suicide Attempts and Deaths

In the ECA study described previously, an association between panic disorder and suicide attempts has been demonstrated. The lifetime rates of suicide attempts in persons with panic disorder and major depression were 20% and 15%, respectively, compared with 6% for persons with another psychiatric disorder and 1% for persons with no psychiatric disorder (Weissman et al. 1989). The lifetime rate of suicide attempts among patients with panic attacks, which were more prevalent than panic disorder, was also high: 12%. Johnson and colleagues (1990) examined rates of suicide attempts among persons with uncomplicated panic disorder or major depression (no other Axis I disorder) to determine whether an increased risk of suicide attempts might be directly related to the high comorbidity between panic disorder and other disorders, such as drug or alcohol abuse or depression. The study found that uncomplicated panic disorder and uncomplicated major depression were uncommon: Only one-fourth of patients had an uncomplicated disorder, but the uncomplicated disorders were still associated with a significantly increased risk of suicide compared with the risk observed in persons with no mental disorder—the increased risk was more than sevenfold. These findings were replicated in a follow-up study on the basis of data gathered by clinically trained interviewers and direct assessment of relatives (Adams and Weissman, submitted for publication). A considerable variability in the patterns of onset of panic disorder, major depression, and suicide attempts, however, precluded any conclusions as to which diagnosis or behavior was a risk factor, which was a consequence, and which was the result of an underlying process. There was some evidence of clustering of the disorders and suicide attempts.

Since these initial observations about the association between panic disorder and suicide attempts were made, other reports have appeared: an epidemiological study by Bland and associates (1988) on more than 3,000 adults living in Edmonton, Canada; studies of alcohol rehabilitation patients by Hasin and co-workers (1988); a 4-year follow-up study (Katschnig 1991) of panic disorder patients from a randomized treatment trial in which 6 of 314 patients made suicide attempts; and other studies (see review by Noyes et al. 1991). However, Beck and others (1991), in a study of panic disorder patients referred to a clinic for cognitive therapy, did not find an increased risk of suicide attempts. It is possible that patients with a history of suicide attempts are less likely to be referred to a clinic exclusively providing psychological treatment.

In Sweden, Allgulander and Lavori (1991) reported excess mortality in patients with anxiety diagnoses on the basis of hospitalization records, case registries, and death certificates. Unfortunately, the available information did not allow for the separation of generalized anxiety disorder from panic disorder. It is likely that a significant sample, perhaps 25% to 40% of the patients with anxiety neurosis diagnoses, would have met criteria for panic disorder. The consistency of the findings in these additional samples lends support to the validity of the initial observations of a relation between panic disorder and suicide attempts, which were based on epidemiological samples.

Quality of Life

As new findings emerged on the efficacy of short-term treatments for panic disorder, attention was directed to long-term treatment for preventing relapse and recurrence and for promoting quality of life. This attention has raised questions about long-term course and medical morbidity, which were discussed previously, and impact on the quality of life of persons with panic disorder, which is discussed later. These questions are similar to those raised on major depression in the 1960s and 1970s. A body of information documenting the social and health impairments associated with depression is now available. Until recently, however, similar information pertinent to panic disorder had not been published; moreover, the psychological and physical effects of panic disorder had been underestimated.

Data from the ECA study were analyzed to gain insight into the social and health consequences of panic disorder compared with those of major depression and of not having a disorder. The conclusion made from the analyses was that panic disorder, like major depression, was associated with self-perception of poor physical and emotional health, increased risk of alcohol abuse, marital and financial problems, and increased medication and emergency room use. For example, in one year, 28% of the patients with panic disorder compared with 11% with major depression and 2% with neither disorder used emergency rooms for an emotional problem. Patients with panic disorder were the most frequent users of emergency rooms when compared with patients with any of the major mental disorders. The prevalence of alcohol abuse was as follows: 27% of patients with panic disorder, 18% of depressed patients, and 11% of those with neither disorder had experienced alcohol problems meeting the DSM-III criteria for alcohol abuse at some point in their lives. Nearly one-third of the patients with panic disorder and a comparable number with major depression perceived their physical health as fair or poor (Markowitz et al. 1989).

Similar analyses were conducted on prevalences of panic attacks in the community to measure their impact on social morbidity and health care utilization (Klerman 1991). Patients with panic attacks not meeting the criteria for panic disorder (because of insufficient symptoms or duration), like those with full-blown panic disorder, often seek help for their symptoms; such symptoms can mimic several medical disorders. Moreover, prevalence of panic attacks is considerably higher (3.6% of the adult population) than that of panic disorder (about 1.5%).

In a similar analysis comparing the social morbidity of panic attacks with that of panic disorder and of other mental disorders, the most important finding was that the effects of panic attacks were intermediate in severity between those of panic disorder and other mental disorders. The major conclusions were that the findings could not be explained by comorbidity of panic attacks with other mental disorders and that panic attacks have clinical significance and are associated with substantial morbidity.

Leon and colleagues (1992) examined the Sheehan Disability Scale (Sheehan 1983), which measures impairment in work, social, and family functioning, in the large worldwide sample of patients seeking treatment of panic disorder in the CNCPS. They found a significant relation between panic symptoms and impairment in functioning.

The HARP study examined quality of life in patients with panic disorder (Massion et al., in press) and had findings similar to those of the ECA study. More than one-quarter of the HARP subjects with panic disorder were receiving public assistance, and only slightly more than one-half (53%) were working full time. Panic disorder was also associated with the subjects' missing work because of mental health problems, marital problems, and high rates of alcohol and other substance abuse or dependence in their lives, and 16% had met criteria for other substance abuse or dependence.

The assessment of quality of life for research purposes is relatively new. Recently, Bech described the difficulties in assessing quality of life associated with specific psychiatric (Bech and Hjortso 1990) and psychosomatic illnesses (Bech 1987, 1990, 1992). He argued that a quality of life assessment should take into account the multidimensional aspect of illness and should be in the context of the patient's own statement. Clearly, such data are currently unavailable for panic disorder.

3   The Origins of Panic Disorder: Etiology and Pathogenesis

S everal theories of etiology and pathogenesis have been suggested to explain the "origins" of panic disorder. (In this chapter, "origins" refers to those empirically demonstrated antecedent factors that influence predisposition or vulnerability to onset of panic disorder.) These theories have also served as a scientific basis for the development of treatment strategies.

In this review, both the etiology and pathogenesis of panic disorder are addressed. Etiology is distinguished from pathogenesis on the basis of the classic medical model; etiology refers to causal factors (why), and pathogenesis refers to the events that occur, particularly at the cellular level, during the development of the disorder (how).

This chapter begins with the most promising etiological theories. It concludes with the most frequently proposed theories of pathogenesis, which are integrated into a single conceptual synthesis that forms a current working hypothesis of panic disorder.

Etiology

During the past 20 years, rapid progress has been made in the field of psychiatry in understanding, diagnosing, and treating many common mental disorders. The advances made in the early characterization of etiological factors underlying panic disorder dramatically highlight this progress. Through a combination of basic neurobiological, molecular genetic, clinical psychobiological, psychopharmacological, and behavioral investigations in both human beings and animals, a clearer understanding of the etiology of panic disorder is emerging.

Biological psychiatrists proposed theories regarding causal factors underlying panic disorder relating to genetically influenced putative abnormalities in neurotransmitter functions. Psychoanalysts and psychologists proposed a number of psychological and developmental theories that emphasized developmental causes. Representative examples from all of these groups of theories are reviewed later.

Genetics and Familial Factors

For many years, a tendency for anxiety disorders to run in families has been observed anecdotally. Several articles published between 1869 and 1948 reported a familial predisposition to anxiety disorders; rates of those disorders in first-degree relatives were reported to be between 14.9% and 18.4%. Since the development of the DSM-III (American Psychiatric Association 1980), family studies have examined the familial aggregation of panic disorder separate from that of other anxiety disorders.

Crowe and colleagues (1983) personally examined 272 first-degree relatives of patients with panic disorder and 262 relatives of control subjects. Whereas the risk of panic disorder was 17.3% in the first-degree relatives of the panic disorder patients, the risk in the relatives of the control subjects was 1.8%. In another study with a similar design, Noyes and colleagues (1986b) found the rates of panic disorder to be 14.9% in the relatives of panic disorder probands and 3.5% in the relatives of matched control subjects. These data are consistent with the premise that panic disorder is a familial disease. The findings from family studies also differentiate panic disorder from other disorders. A review of such findings can be found in Chapter 4.

Two twin studies on panic disorder have now been reported. In a small sample of twins with panic-like symptoms selected from psychiatric facilities in Norway, Torgersen (1983) found a concordance rate in monozygotic (MZ) twins of 31% (4 of 13); no concordance was noted (0 of 16) in dizygotic (DZ) twins. In a recent large population-based sample of female-female pairs, Kendler and colleagues (1992a) found modestly higher concordance rates for panic disorder in MZ (24%) versus DZ (11%) twins. Applying a multifactorial threshold model, they estimated the heritability of a liability to panic disorder at 35% to 40%; the full results of the study have not yet been reported. No adoption studies of panic disorder have been published to date. (For additional information on twin studies, see Chapter 4.)

Family studies have begun to address possible relationships among the familial factors that influence panic disorder and those that affect the risk of other major psychiatric disorders. Current evidence regarding a possible familial relationship between panic disorder and major depression is still inconclusive. In two studies, no excess risk for major depression was found in relatives of persons with panic disorder versus relatives of matched control subjects (Crowe et al. 1983; Noyes et al. 1986b). These findings are supported by a new and as yet unpublished family study by Weissman (in press). However, Leckman and colleagues (1983) found that patients with both major depression and panic disorder had relatives who were at increased risk of both disorders compared with relatives of control subjects. Noyes and colleagues (1986) investigated a possible familial interrelationship between panic disorder and agoraphobia. Whereas there was some evidence for shared familial factors, there was also evidence that these disorders were not, from a familial perspective, the same condition. In their population-based sample of twins, Kendler and colleagues (1992a) found evidence that panic disorder with phobic avoidance or agoraphobia could, from a familial-genetic perspective, be considered a severe variant of uncomplicated panic disorder.

Recent interest in the mode of transmission of panic disorder has begun to yield useful information. Complex segregation analysis on one modest-size sample of pedigrees has supported the hypothesis that the familial aggregation of panic disorder is due to a single dominant major locus of relatively high penetration (Pauls et al. 1980). However, this finding is not fully consistent with the results of the one population-based twin study, which suggested that the heritability of panic disorder is considerably lower than that predicted from the high-density pedigrees. This discrepancy could be due to several factors, including differences between clinical and epidemiological samples of persons with panic disorder.

The promising results of the twin studies indicating that panic disorder is likely to be a genetic disease and the availability of molecular genetic techniques have fueled the application of these techniques to the study of panic disorder in the past 5 years. Initial positive evidence of genetic linkage to alpha-haptoglobin from Crowe and colleagues (1987), however, could not be replicated by the same researchers (1990). The consistency of the previous family data has been so encouraging that a number of research teams worldwide are conducting molecular genetic linkage studies in panic disorder. These groups are in the process of identifying informative families with high concentrations of panic disorder across generations.

Psychological Theories:
Psychodynamic and Psychoanalytic Theories

Several psychodynamic theories have been proposed to explain why anxiety states develop. According to the classic theory of anxiety, signal anxiety is generated by contemporary experiences similar to previous events that threaten to overwhelm the ego and awaken unresolved unconscious conflicts. Alternatively, panic apprehension may be conceived as the emergence of deeply rooted unconscious conflicts, primarily aggressive in character, that originated in traumatic experiences in early childhood.

In his early work, Freud (1895/1940) made a clear distinction between anxiety neurosis, which he described in terms that closely parallel the current DSM-III-R (American Psychiatric Association 1987) definition of panic disorder, and psychoneurotic states. He viewed anxiety neurosis, along with neurasthenia, as "actual neuroses" with a somatic etiology, requiring a nonpsychological treatment (i.e., a change in sexual behavior). Psychoneuroses (e.g., phobias, obsessive-compulsive disorder, or hysteria), in which anxiety was psychically bound, arose from psychic conflict caused by early developmental traumas and therefore was accessible through psychoanalytic treatment. Freud never fully abandoned his view of actual neuroses, referring in *Inhibitions, Symptoms and Anxiety* (Freud 1926/1948) to one type of anxiety that "was involuntary, automatic and always justified on economic grounds" (p. 162). In this work, however, Freud revised his theory of anxiety, describing it as an intrapsychic response to psychologically meaningful danger. In addition to autonomic anxiety, he described a second type of anxiety that signaled the ego to institute a defense against the danger of emergent forbidden wishes. The new theory of anxiety as a response to danger led Freud to delineate a series of developmentally significant fears: helplessness, separation, castration, and finally, in its most mature form, superego anxiety. Many psychoanalysts, using the new theory, came to view any form of anxiety as secondary to the emergence of forbidden unconscious wishes, requiring a psychoanalytic approach. This view, however, ignored Freud's proviso that under certain conditions, such as acute trauma, automatic anxiety could be expressed as panic.

Currently available empirical data that support the separation of panic disorder from generalized anxiety disorder have not affected the psychoanalytic view of the etiology of anxiety. Unfortunately, as of now, no distinction is currently made in psychodynamic theory between panic attacks, panic disorder, and generalized anxiety states.

Psychological Theories: Learning and Behavior Theories

For many decades, anxiety disorders have been considered within the framework of learning theories, including classical conditioning and the two-way avoidance learning theory (Hollander et al. 1988). Most of the attention focused on anxiety disorders has been paid to phobic states, particularly agoraphobia. However, until recently, panic attacks per se have not received special attention within the learning theory paradigm. In behavioral theories, panic attacks have been generally considered to be a very severe or intense form of pathological anxiety and not a distinct disease.

Learning theory is derived primarily from studies of learning in animals; its clinical applications are supported by evidence from studies of the efficacy of behavior therapy in reducing anxiety and avoidance. Learning theories are more successful at explaining how panic attacks recur and how agoraphobia develops after a panic attack than in explaining the etiology of a first panic attack. After an original spontaneous panic attack, further situation-specific panic attacks occur through conditioning in those situations in which anxiety has already been experienced. Phobic avoidance develops as patients seek to prevent further panic attacks and then prevents the reconditioning of fear of responses through extinction. In terms of learning theory, panic attacks that occur in phobic situations are markedly severe forms of phobic anxiety.

Learning theory considers spontaneous panic attacks a particularly severe form of anticipatory anxiety in which the panic attack occurs as the patient thinks about or visualizes phobic situations. Although this sequence is described by many patients whose panic attacks appeared at first to be spontaneous, it is not always the case. For this reason, a second explanation has been proposed; namely, that panic attacks arise when anxiety is conditioned to internal stimuli. For example, if anxiety is accompanied by palpitations, an increase in heart rate (e.g., after exercise or in response to everyday stressful events) will lead to conditioned anxiety. Following this hypothesis, panic attacks have been treated by deconditioning the anxiety response to palpitations (or other symptoms of panic attack) by repeatedly inducing panic attacks through the use of inhaled carbon dioxide. When this procedure is repeated, it results in a desensitization to the internal stimuli and a diminished anxiety response. Good results have been reported from this approach (Griez and Van den Hout 1986), which suggests that conditioned responses of the type described here are potentially important.

Psychological Theories: Cognitive Theory

The cognitive theory of panic disorder originated by Clark (1986) proposes that panic attacks develop when a person misinterprets the significance of certain bodily sensations. According to this model (reviewed by Craske and Barlow 1988), the cognitive misinterpretation is that the bodily sensations are forerunners of an impending medical emergency. For example, palpitations are misinterpreted as a sign of a heart attack. This misinterpretation leads, understandably, to heightened anxiety, which in turn leads to greater autonomic arousal and more pronounced palpitations. In this way, the original misinterpretation sets up a positive feedback loop that results in rapidly escalating anxiety, culminating in a panic attack. This hypothesis differs from the conditioning theory reviewed previously, which proposes an automatic conditioned association without a cognitive component. When panic attacks arise from cognitive misinterpretations, the learning mechanisms discussed previously may also lead to the development of additional symptoms by conditioning panic attacks to occur in response to specific external situations. In turn, avoidance may develop, in which case the condition becomes panic disorder with agoraphobia. Thus, the conditioning and cognitive theories of panic are complementary, not exclusive.

The cognitive hypothesis is supported by considerable evidence. Reports from patients with panic disorder confirm that thoughts of imminent danger accompany panic attacks (Hibbert 1984; Ottaviani and Beck 1987). In panic disorder patients, an increase in the bodily sensations that are thought to provoke panic attacks leads to greater anxiety (Ehlers et al. 1988). Also, reducing relevant misinterpretations diminishes the effect of agents that otherwise provoke panic attacks (Clark et al. 1988). Further support for the cognitive hypothesis comes from the effects of cognitive-behavioral therapy (described in detail in Chapter 5). Briefly, cognitive-behavioral treatment that targets the reduction of misinterpretations leads to the reduction of panic attacks.

It is not known why some patients misinterpret bodily sensations catastrophically and develop panic attacks, whereas others do not. In some cases, the mistaken beliefs seem to originate from the knowledge that the patient has about an illness of a significant other (e.g., about heart disease in a relative). In other cases, no such simple explanation is available, and the beliefs may possibly have developed at the first panic attack or attacks: For example, the first attacks of panic may have been mistaken for and treated as cardiac emergencies, and the misinterpretations may then have become maintaining factors for future panic attacks rather than merely being a predisposing cause of the first attack. The long-term beneficial effects of cognitive therapy (see Chapter 5) suggest that cognitive factors are both predisposing and maintaining factors for panic attacks. Because relapse is uncommon when cognitive factors have been modified successfully, such factors may play an important role in the etiology of panic disorder.

Developmental Theories: Childhood Separation Anxiety

A relationship has been proposed between childhood separation anxiety and other psychopathological conditions, such as overanxious disorder, school phobia, adult panic disorder, and agoraphobia. Several studies suggested that separation anxiety and other childhood anxiety disorders are early forms of panic disorder (Moreau and Weissman 1992). However, Perugi and colleagues (1988) found that 60% of patients diagnosed with panic disorder and agoraphobia had histories of school phobia in childhood, whereas no childhood separation anxiety was noted for uncomplicated panic disorder patients. Thus, it is unclear whether separation anxiety is associated with panic or with agoraphobia. Longitudinal studies of children with anxiety disorders and family studies examining transmission of anxiety disorders across the generations may sort this out.

Developmental Theories: Childhood Behavioral Inhibition

Research in child development (Biederman 1990; Kagan and Snidman 1991; Kagan et al. 1988) and developmental psychopathology (Rosenbaum et al. 1992) has provided intriguing information on the potential developmental antecedents of panic and anxiety disorders and, at the same time, has suggested the role of genetic factors. Children whose parents have been diagnosed with panic disorder are significantly more likely to be classified as behaviorally inhibited (i.e., exhibiting fear and withdrawal in novel or unfamiliar situations). Conversely, parents of behaviorally inhibited children have markedly higher rates of anxiety disorders.

Developmental Theories: Parental Child-Rearing Attitudes and Behavior

A few observers have found that patients with panic disorder describe their parents as overprotective, restricting, controlling, critical, frightening, and rejecting. Tucker (1956) found that 77 of 100 phobic patients without a control group contrast reported overprotection and overcriticism by parents as well as a lack of parental affection. Some confirmation of these observations has come from more systematic studies that assess perception of parents with questionnaires, which have been found to be highly reliable and valid. Parker (1979), using the Parental Bonding Instrument (Parker et al. 1979), found that a group of patients with social phobia and patients with agoraphobia viewed their parents as significantly less caring and more overprotective than did control subjects. This finding was later confirmed by Silove (1986) for a group of agoraphobic patients compared with a control group. Arrindell and colleagues (1983), with a more detailed questionnaire, the Egna Minnen Betraffande Uppfostran (My Memories of Upbringing [Perris et al. 1980]), found that agoraphobic patients viewed both parents as having significantly less emotional warmth and their mothers as being more rejecting than did control subjects. It should be emphasized that these theories are based on retrospective reports by adults, some but not all of whom may have had panic disorder. Direct observational studies are needed to confirm these theories.

Conclusion

Although some of the hypotheses that have been proposed to explain the etiology of panic have only modest empirical foundations, many have had heuristic value and have spawned a large number of studies on panic disorder. Although no etiology for panic disorder has been definitively identified, many lines of investigation have generated promising data elucidating some potential etiological factors.

Pathogenesis and Pathophysiology: Experimental Models and Biological Theories

Current biologically based theories for the pathogenesis of panic disorder have been drawn from a number of experimental models and observations. This section presents the most important models and observations, followed by some of the theories that have been advanced and relevant supportive data.

Provocation and Challenge Studies

To study the pathogenetic processes that occur when a person has a panic attack, researchers have devised methods to induce panic attacks. Several of these methods are described next.

Sodium lactate. Pitts and McClure's (1967) early finding that sodium lactate could provoke panic anxiety has often been replicated in patients with panic disorder. Today the lactate provocation test is considered one of the most robust indicators of an underlying biological basis for panic disorder. Several studies, but not all, have found the lactate challenge to be reasonably sensitive and specific. Interestingly, lactate precipitation of panic attacks can be eliminated or diminished by pretreatment with imipramine, a therapeutically effective medication. The panicogenic property of lactate and the elimination of the panic response with imipramine have been demonstrated in macaque monkeys and human beings. The mechanism of action of lactate provocation of panic attacks is still under investigation. It has been suggested that lactate acts on the locus ceruleus of the brain stem and that imipramine increases the threshold for lactate induction of panic anxiety.

Carbon dioxide, yohimbine, and other agents. The inhalation of carbon dioxide and the oral administration of yohimbine, an alpha$_2$-receptor antagonist, may also precipitate panic attacks in panic disorder patients in laboratory settings. Other pharmacological agents, including caffeine, isoproterenol, norepinephrine, flumazenil (a benzodiazepine [BZ] antagonist), and cholecystokinin (a neuropeptide), have also precipitated panic attacks in panic disorder patients.

The availability of provocative agents with different pharmacological profiles has been extremely useful in studying the characteristics of panic attacks as well as in elucidating the potential pathophysiological mechanisms in the brain that underlie these attacks. As yet, however, challenge studies have not been useful in the diagnosis and clinical management of panic disorder.

Neuroendocrine and Other Biological Markers

The investigation of various neuroendocrine challenges in panic disorder has been useful in identifying the neurotransmitter system abnormalities that may underlie panic disorder. Generally, the patterns of response in patients with panic disorder are different from those of depressed patients. Other biological markers studied in panic disorder include monoamine oxidase, serotonin uptake, alpha2-adrenoceptor and 3H-imipramine receptors in platelets, and serotonin and norepinephrine metabolism. The use of this research strategy has produced some interesting but not strongly confirmatory data in support of the various hypotheses that propose that neurotransmitter abnormalities play a role in panic disorder.

Animal Models of Anxiety and Arousal States

Animal models such as Maudsley and Roman rodent strains are available for the study of generalized arousal and anxiety states. However, there are no good animal models for panic attacks-panic disorder per se. Nevertheless, investigations in a number of different animal models of anxiety have implicated various brain structures as being heavily involved in intense arousal-anxiety states. These brain structures, which include the septal region, the amygdaloid nuclei, the hippocampus, and the parahippocampal gyrus, are loosely grouped into the limbic system (septohippocampal region), which has been identified as being activated or abnormal during pathological anxiety states (Gray 1982). Data from these basic studies in animals have helped delineate the potential brain regions that play a role in anxiety disorders in human beings, allowing directed scientific inquiry to focus on specific brain structures in patients with panic disorder.

Functional Brain Imaging Studies

With new functional neuroimaging technology such as positron-emission tomography (PET), it is now possible on a routine basis to observe the living human brain while it is in the process of functioning. Thus, investigators have been able to observe changes in the brains of panic disorder patients. Specifically, significant abnormal cerebral blood flow patterns have been identified and measured in the parahippo-campal and hippocampal regions of the brain in panic disorder (Nordahl et al. 1990). The observations from PET studies have been on the same regions of the brain that had previously been found to be abnormal in animal model studies. The combination of neurochemical and anatomical studies in animals and functional neuroimaging studies in panic disorder patients has begun to define a characteristic neuroanatomy of panic and anxiety disorders in humans.

Nocturnal Panic Attacks

During the past few years, Mellman and Uhde (1989, 1990) observed that approximately 69% of panic disorder patients report the occurrence of panic attacks during sleep and one-third of patients report that panic attacks during sleep are recurrent. Polysomnographic studies have identified the following sleep abnormalities in these patients: increased sleep latency, decreased sleep time, and decreased sleep efficiency. On nights when panic attacks occurred during sleep, an increase in rapid eye movement (REM) latency was also noted.

Neurochemical and Neurotransmitter Theories

Neurochemical, neuropsychopharmacological, neuroanatomical, and cellular and molecular biological studies have identified consistent abnormalities in the following three specific central nervous system (CNS) neurotransmitter systems in persons with panic anxiety: the noradrenergic system, the serotonergic system, and the BZ receptor and gamma-aminobutyric acid (GABA) system. The identification and study of these neurotransmitter systems have generated several theories related to abnormal transmitter function, which are described next.

Noradrenergic theory.   It has been hypothesized that increased activity or reactivity of the noradrenergic neurotransmitter system either causes or is related to panic anxiety. The initial evidence for this hypothesis is based on animal studies in which activation of neurons in the locus ceruleus, the primary source of noradrenergic (norepinephrine-releasing) neurons in the brain, consistently produced arousal and anxiety states (Gray 1982). In addition, investigations in clinical populations have found increased levels of norepinephrine and its metabolite 3-methoxy-4-hydroxyphenylglycol (MHPG) in the cerebrospinal fluid of panic disorder patients (Charney et al. 1984). Patients with panic disorder were also observed to have increased plasma concentrations of epinephrine and MHPG (Villacres et al. 1987). Further support for this hypothesis has been provided by challenge studies with specific alpha-adrenergic-receptor antagonist and agonist agents. Challenges with yohimbine, a norepinephrine antagonist, result in increased panic anxiety and MHPG levels (Charney et al. 1984). Reciprocally, challenges with clonidine, a norepinephrine agonist, appear to decrease anxiety, MHPG, and growth hormone responses in panic disorder (Charney and Heninger 1986). Finally, both tricyclic antidepressants (TCAs) and monoamine oxidase inhibitors (MAOIs) were found to inhibit activation of the locus ceruleus by corticotropin-releasing factor during stressful states. This latter observation suggests that one of the neuropharmacological mechanisms mediating the therapeutic effect of these antidepressants in panic disorder is related to their effects in the locus ceruleus.

Serotonergic theory. It has been also hypothesized that increased serotonin (5-HT) neurotransmission may cause or be correlated with panic anxiety. Supporting this hypothesis is the finding that challenges with m-chloro-phenyl-piperazine, a 5-HT agonist, increase both anxiety and the cortisol response in panic disorder patients (Kahn et al. 1988). Further, BZ anxiolytics have been shown to increase 5-HT turnover in serotonergic neurons that arise from the raphe nuclei (Nutt and Cowen 1987).

Buspirone, which acts as an agonist on the presynaptic 5-HT$_{1A}$ somatic dendritic autoreceptors to dampen serotonergic neuronal activity, has proved to be an effective anxiolytic in generalized anxiety disorder. Finally, TCAs, which are therapeutically effective in panic disorder, also act to downregulate the same 5-HT autoreceptors (Goodwin et al. 1985).

Benzodiazepine gamma-aminobutyric acid receptor theory. Currently, the strongest supporting evidence characterizing the pathogenesis of panic disorder entails the relationship among the BZ receptor, the inhibitory neurotransmitter GABA, the GABA-A receptor, and the capacity to regulate the patency of the neuronal chloride ion channel (i.e., the BZ receptor-GABA-A-Cl⁻-ionophore complex). This macromolecular complex is the site of action of the BZs, which make up one of the established classes of anxiolytic medications. Also, the distribution of this receptor complex in the human brain roughly parallels that of the CNS regions previously identified as being involved in pathological anxiety states in animals and by PET in humans.

There are several working hypotheses involving the BZ-GABA receptor complex. First, it has been hypothesized that panic disorder may be caused by an abnormality, possibly subsensitivity or underactivation of the BZ receptor. In support of this hypothesis is the evidence that patients with panic disorder patients manifest decreased BZ receptor sensitivity (Roy-Byrne et al. 1990) and that flumazenil, a BZ receptor antagonist, can stimulate panic attacks in such patients (Nutt 1990).

Abnormal endogenous ligand theory. Recently, the characterization of the BZ receptor has initiated aggressive scientific investigation to identify putative endogenous or naturally occurring ligands that might be present in the brains of patients with panic disorder. The first of two hypotheses is that panic disorder is caused by an excess of an abnormal endogenous ligand or ligands that are anxiogenic or anxiety producing in their effects on the BZ-GABA-A-Cl⁻-ionophore complex. An example of one such putative ligand is diazepam binding inhibitor (Barbaccia et al. 1986).

The second hypothesis, the converse of the first, proposes that panic disorder is due to a deficit in naturally occurring ligands that are anxiolytic or antianxiogenic in their effect on this same macromolecular complex. Consistent with this hypothesis is the identification of two naturally occurring pregnane steroids—3 alpha, 5 alpha-tetrahydroxycorticosterone and 3 alpha-hydroxy-5 alpha-dihydroprogesterone—that interact with the BZ-GABA-A-Cl⁻-ionophore complex producing potent hypnotic-anxiolytic effects. In addition, the exogenous pregnane steroid, alphaxalone, has also been demonstrated to reduce anxiety behavior in a rodent model of anxiety (Britton et al. 1991). These very interesting findings may eventually lead to the identification and development of a new class of antianxiety drugs. More immediately, they provide a potentially profound insight into the pathophysiology of panic disorder.

Panic Disorder as a Variant of a Convulsive Disorder

The clinical similarities between certain features of panic attacks such as paroxysmal onset and altered states of awareness (apprehension, depersonalization, and derealization) and the demonstration of abnormalities in cerebral blood flow in the temporal lobes, with their important connections to the limbic system, suggest that panic disorder may be a seizure-like disorder. However, that view is not supported by electroencephalographic (EEG) recordings from panic disorder patients, although scalp EEG techniques may not be suitable to demonstrate involvement of deep brain structures. Moreover, carbamazepine has not proved to be an effective antipanic drug. Thus, there is little consistent empirical evidence to date to support the hypothesis that panic disorder is a variant of convulsive disorder.

A Current Working Hypothesis of Panic Disorder

The most conservative interpretation and synthesis of all the data primarily from biological studies, and to a smaller extent from psychological studies, into a working hypothetical model of the pathogenesis and pathophysiology of panic disorder is as follows: Patients with panic disorder may have inherited a genetic vulnerability or constitutional predisposition to experience spontaneous panic attacks. This propensity to panic attacks may first manifest early in childhood in the form of behavioral inhibition (shyness) and then later in adult life as panic disorder. The elaboration of the putative genetic diathesis in panic disorder patients may result from the cumulative perturbation of arousing stressful environmental events (see Chapter 4). In other words, a true diathesis-stress model in a reciprocal brain-environment interactional framework may be operating.

Central to the general hypothetical model of the pathogenesis of panic disorder are the following potential brain mechanisms: The core feature in the development of panic disorder is an initial intense activation of the septohippocampal region of the brain. This activation in turn is discharged through efferent pathways to the cortex (including prefrontal areas), hypothalamus, thalamus, and anterior pituitary. The resultant changes in these latter brain structures are hypothesized to generate the signs and symptoms that are characteristic of panic attacks. Furthermore, the septohippocampal region can be activated in several important ways. First, activation can occur spontaneously within the septohippocampal structures themselves. Second, septohippocampal activation can result from increased input from noradrenergic neurons arising in the locus ceruleus. Third, activation of this region can occur from the serotonergic neurons arising from cell bodies in the raphe nuclei of the midbrain. Finally, and perhaps most important, a dysfunction (e.g., a deficit) in the BZ receptors can also result in a diminution of the inhibitory influence of GABA directly on the septohippocampal region and on the cell bodies and neurons derived from both the locus ceruleus (norepinephrine) and the raphe nuclei (serotonin). This latter component of the hypothesis is compelling given the broad inhibitory influence of GABA on each of the brain regions that appears to be involved in panic disorder. There appears to be a converging confluence of evidence that strongly suggests that, in the not-too-distant future, a clearer, more concise, and fully substantiated pathophysiological model of panic disorder will be available.

Pathogenesis and Pathophysiology: Psychological and Psychosocial Theories

Life Events as Precipitants

Many studies indicate that significant life events precede the onset of panic disorder (Faravelli 1985; Last et al. 1984; Roy-Byrne et al. 1986). However, it is not known whether those events exert their influence through a psychological mechanism (evoking catastrophic cognition as a form of maladaptive coping response) or through the provocation of a disorder in which the primary etiology is based on a genetic predisposition.

Faravelli (1985), with a more systematic approach, found a higher number of life events in patients with a first panic attack compared with healthy control subjects in the 12 months preceding the onset of panic attacks, noting that "both loss events and threatening events seem to play a role" (p. 105) in the onset of panic anxiety. In addition, Roy-Byrne and colleagues (1986) found that panic patients reported significantly more life events in the 12 months preceding their first panic attack compared with control subjects. The patients also reported significantly more subjective distress about their life events compared with control subjects, and events were viewed by the patients in comparison with the control subjects as more undesirable and uncontrollable and having caused extreme lowering of self-esteem.

Interpretation is made more difficult because response to a life event depends on the meaning of the event to the person to whom it happens as well as its objective magnitude and impact. Thus, a panic attack could arise when an event is interpreted as a specific threat to a person, and the event may also create a much greater effect in persons with a predisposition to panic anxiety than in others not afflicted with panic disorder.

Predisposing Factors in Adolescent and Adult Personality

Studies of personality have not permitted the separation of patients with panic disorder from those comorbidly afflicted with both panic disorder and agoraphobia. This distinction is potentially important because some of the personality characteristics identified in patients with agoraphobia may be more specifically related to the development of avoidance behavior than to the development of panic attacks. Several authors suggested that patients with panic disorder and agoraphobia were unassertive, fearful, and dependent before the disorder began. The character traits described in these patients could be relevant both to the tendency to develop anxiety under stress and to the propensity to avoidance behavior. For example, Marks (1970) reported that most people with agoraphobia have a premorbid personality that he described as soft, passive, anxious, shy, and dependent. Klein (1964) reported that approximately half of his patients were "fearful and dependent as children, with marked separation anxiety and difficulty in adjusting in school" (p. 405). Torgersen (1986) found a significantly higher rate of chronic anxiety reported in childhood in a group of patients with panic disorder compared with a group of patients with generalized anxiety disorder.

Other researchers suggested that panic disorder patients have difficulty tolerating anger, but these reports are not based on empirical evidence. It was also suggested that phobic anxiety is associated with aggressive impulses and that the anxiety is reduced in the presence of a companion because the patient is unconsciously relieved that the aggressive impulses have not harmed the person. Korn and associates (1992) described four cases in which anger was believed to precipitate panic attacks. Although this sequence of events can be observed occasionally, there is no evidence that it is related to specific personality traits. Instead, the sequence may be related to a more generalized emotional arousal that culminates in persons with this predisposition.

4 Validity of Panic Disorder as a Nosological Entity

The establishment of the validity of panic disorder as a nosological category distinct from other categories remains controversial. As noted before, panic disorder was included in the *International Classification of Diseases* (ICD) diagnostic system for the first time in the 10th edition (ICD-10; World Health Organization 1992) and, in the United States, has been in the *Diagnostic and Statistical Manual of Mental Disorders* (DSM) only since 1980 (American Psychiatric Association 1980). Despite this recent official recognition, a large body of empirical data, much of which has been presented earlier in this review, has been generated relevant to the issue of the validity of the disorder. This chapter organizes the data relevant to the question of validity.

A useful heuristic framework for examining and establishing the validity of a diagnostic entity was presented by E. Robins and Guze (1970). To establish diagnostic validity, they recommended that the following five areas be examined: clinical description, laboratory studies, delimitation from other disorders, follow-up studies, and family studies.

Clinical description includes the clinical picture of the disorder, emphasizing aspects that distinguish it from other disorders. Laboratory studies can include, for example, biochemical, radiological, and psychological studies and must be objective, reliable, and reproducible. Delimitation from other disorders simply means demonstrating the separateness of a particular illness from other illnesses. Follow-up studies demonstrate that a disorder is associated with a distinct outcome pattern. Family studies show characteristic prevalences of a disorder in families and represent one method of demonstrating delimitation from other disorders. The procedure proposed by E. Robins and Guze is similar to the two stages in the identification of a mental disorder as a diagnostic entity proposed by Foulds and Hope (1968) and demonstrated empirically by Priest (Priest 1976; Priest and Laffont 1992).

Clinical Description of Panic Disorder

The clinical description of panic disorder is striking. Its central symptom is the panic attack: a sudden, unprecipitated episode of symptoms such as shortness of breath, dizziness, tachycardia, chest pain, and fear of dying. Agoraphobia, often associated with panic disorder, is an intense fear of being alone in a place or unable to get help if a panic attack were to occur there. This fear often leads a person to become housebound or unable to go places unless accompanied by someone whom that person trusts. Some common agoraphobic situations include being in a crowd, driving a car alone, and being home alone.

Currently, the number of panic attacks and how frequently they must occur to meet the criteria for panic disorder is under debate. However, there is little disagreement about the specific criteria that make up a panic attack. Whether or not specific criteria should be weighted has not been resolved.

Important issues relevant to panic disorder include the significance of limited symptom panic attacks (i.e., attacks that do not meet all the criteria for a panic attack). Other areas of interest are the significance of a single panic attack or extremely infrequent panic attacks, the rapidity and intensity of onset necessary to distinguish an attack as a panic attack, and the separation of a precipitated panic attack (e.g., an attack that occurs on confronting a snake or being in an elevator) from an unprecipitated panic attack.

Laboratory Studies

A number of agents can precipitate panic attacks in the laboratory. Pitts and McClure (1967) demonstrated that sodium lactate can provoke panic attacks in susceptible patients. Since that time, a number of other investigators reproduced that finding and demonstrated that a variety of other substances, including carbon dioxide (Fyer et al. 1987a), yohimbine (Charney et al. 1987; Henauer et al. 1984), caffeine (Charney et al. 1985), isoproterenol (Tainey et al. 1984), and noradrenaline (Tainey et al. 1984), can precipitate panic attacks.

Positron-emission tomography and magnetic resonance imaging studies demonstrated the existence of abnormalities that are somewhat characteristic of patients with panic disorder but are not found in those with simple fear.

Delimitation From Other Disorders

Evidence from epidemiological community surveys, family studies, and twin studies supports the separation of panic disorder from other psychiatric disorders, particularly generalized anxiety disorder. The available epidemiological data are summarized in the following paragraph. Findings from family studies and twin studies have been previously reviewed.

Modern diagnostic criteria were used in at least seven recently completed community surveys, and those studies provided some information on the prevalence rates of various anxiety disorders in the community (Angst et al. 1987; Canino et al. 1987; Murphy 1986; Regier et al. 1984; Uhlenhuth et al. 1983; Weissman 1988; Wittchen 1986a). The largest of these studies was the National Institute of Mental Health Epidemiologic Catchment Area survey, which was conducted between 1980 and 1984. This study, conducted independently at five sites in the United States, made use of the Diagnostic Interview Schedule (L. N. Robins et al. 1981), a forerunner of the DSM-III diagnostic criteria. On the basis of data from several of the studies, 2.5 of 100 to 8.1 of 100 persons met the criteria for generalized anxiety disorder in any one year. These rates were slightly higher in women and may be higher in the lower socioeconomic classes. Only about 1% of persons (0.4 of 100 to 1.6 of 100) met the criteria for panic disorder in any 1- to 12-month period. The rates were higher in persons aged 25 to 44 years and in those living in urban areas. Onset occurred in the middle of the fourth decade of life (the mid-30s). There was no strong correlation with race or education.

Evidence for a distinction between panic disorder and generalized anxiety disorder on the basis of epidemiological data shows that the two disorders are associated with different prevalence rates. The current prevalence rates of generalized anxiety disorder, which range from 2.5% to 8%, are considerably higher than those of panic disorder. Additionally, rates of generalized anxiety disorder are consistently higher in women than in men. The current prevalence of panic disorder is about 1%, and the sex ratios vary.

Although the two disorders undoubtedly overlap in some persons and some cases of generalized anxiety disorder may develop into panic disorder, the epidemiological data, when complemented with the data from family and twin studies described in Chapter 3, thus far support the separation of these disorders.

Follow-Up Studies

A review of five studies conducted before the modern era of panic disorder treatment (approximately 1940 to 1960) revealed that about one-third of patients were well or much improved at follow-up, up to 10 years after they were initially studied. Approximately one-third had moderate symptoms, and one-third were unchanged or worse. Eight naturalistic follow-up studies (over periods of 1 to 8 years) of patients with panic disorder have been conducted in the past decade. Compared with the earlier studies, the modern studies show substantial reductions in unimproved patients (from one-third to one-sixth) and modest changes in other outcome measures. (See also Chapter 2, which discusses these studies from the perspective of the data they provide about the long-term course of panic disorder.)

HARP, a prospective, naturalistic study, reported on 309 patients with DSM-III-R (American Psychiatric Association 1987) panic disorder with or without agoraphobia (Keller et al., in press). One year after study entry, subjects with uncomplicated panic disorder had a .37 probability of having full remission (eight or more consecutive weeks with minimal symptoms), and subjects with panic disorder with agoraphobia had only a .16 probability of remission. However, more than one-third of those subjects had relapsed within 10 months of their remissions.

Among the modern treatment era studies is the Cross-National Collaborative Panic Study, in which 367 patients were observed for up to 6 years after a clinical trial for panic disorder. In that study, the course of panic disorder was severe and chronic in nearly one-fifth of patients, whereas one-third of the patients recovered and stayed well, and the course of illness in the remainder was intermediate (Katschnig 1991).

Family Studies and Twin Studies

Family and twin studies already reviewed have supported the notion that panic disorder is a distinct nosological entity. They have demonstrated that panic disorder is highly familial and is distinct from generalized anxiety disorder.

5

Treatments for Panic Anxiety: Research Findings

General Considerations

There is a close relation between advances in clinical, epidemiological, and psychobiological research on panic disorder (see Chapters 2 and 3) and progress in treatment of the disorder. Careful and reliable descriptions of clinical phenomena allowed better delineation of inclusion and exclusion criteria for clinical trial design. As evidence for the efficacy and safety of both psychopharmacological and psychological treatments has accumulated, new controversies have emerged. In the 1970s and early 1980s, the paramount issues were dosage and the conduction of studies for establishing the short-term efficacy and safety of treatments for symptomatic and disabled persons with panic disorder, particularly those studies that would demonstrate the ability of treatments to block panic attacks.

By the mid-1980s, compounds from three classes of psychopharmacological agents had been demonstrated to be effective against panic disorder in placebo-controlled clinical trials: tricyclic antidepressants (TCAs), monoamine oxidase inhibitors (MAOIs), and some benzodiazepines. At the same time, several psychological treatments, particularly behavioral and cognitive treatments, were developed and evaluated.

Psychopharmacological Treatments

Historical Background

From antiquity to the present day, persons from many cultures have used alcohol for nonspecific tranquilization as well as for other purposes. In the early 20th century, bromides were used as sedatives followed by barbiturates and then meprobamate. Those agents, in turn, were replaced by the benzodiazepines, which represent the standard anxiolytics in use today. Through the late 19th and early 20th centuries, many medications have been used to treat panic disorder: opiates, chloral hydrate, alcohol, and substances derived from botanical herbal sources. In the absence of systematic studies, the efficacy of these medications cannot be supported.

The era of modern psychopharmacology in the 1950s permitted the acceleration of the search for effective treatments for anxiety. Beginning in the 1950s, large numbers of psychopharmacological compounds were investigated for possible therapeutic efficacy for what would now be called panic disorder.

Interpretation of these studies from the perspective of the post-DSM-III (American Psychiatric Association 1980) era is difficult because few of them separated panic attacks and panic disorder from other forms of anxiety. Patients were diagnosed as having "anxiety neurosis" or "anxiety states" or characterized with similar nonspecific diagnostic terms. Few studies described the specific diagnostic criteria used, thereby making it impossible for future researchers to replicate the findings. However, it is likely that a substantial number of patients in studies of antianxiety agents in the 1960s and 1970s had what today would be called panic disorder.

Among the compounds investigated were barbiturates, phenothiazines, and other antipsychotic agents; beta-adrenergic blocking agents, particularly propranolol, meprobamate, and other nonbarbiturate sedatives; sedative-hypnotics; and most notably, the conventional benzodiazepines. Although the quality of the clinical research was variable, most of the studies produced little therapeutic success, and, in the cases of the phenothiazines and the barbiturates, adverse effects overshadowed any limited antianxiety benefit.

The conventional wisdom among experienced psychopharmacologists, such as Sheehan and Klein in the 1970s and early 1980s, was that benzodiazepine tranquilizers did not provide therapeutic benefit in the dosages used. However, the persistence of many patients in taking those medications suggested that, although benefit may have been limited, benzodiazepine tranquilizers were still perceived by patients as useful. An alternative interpretation has been proposed by Lader (1992) and others, who referred to the concept of "therapeutic levels of dependence," suggesting that the persistence by patients in the use of the drugs at clinically insufficient dosages is indicative of dependence.

Two developments resulting in more specific and efficacious treatment for panic disorder occurred in the 1960s and 1970s: studies of MAOIs and studies of TCAs. In the United Kingdom, a number of investigators explored the value of MAOIs in atypical depression, phobic anxiety, agoraphobia, and anxiety states. The diagnostic term "panic disorder" was not used in studies conducted in the United Kingdom, but panic attacks were frequently reported. Initial studies were with iproniazid in the treatment of what was diagnosed as "atypical depression" (Sargant 1962; West and Dally 1959). Studies with phenelzine followed (Kelly et al. 1970; Tyrer et al. 1973).

At the same time in the United States, Fink, Klein, and their associates reported the efficacy of imipramine in blocking panic attacks in a randomized trial comparing imipramine and chlorpromazine in hospitalized patients with a wide range of diagnostic conditions (Fink et al. 1965; Klein 1964; Klein and Fink 1962). Klein further assessed the efficacy of imipramine in a series of controlled studies (Zitrin et al. 1980, 1983). He also revived interest in the lactate provocation phenomenon first described by Pitts and McClure (1967), building on Kelley's observation that MAOIs blocked lactate-provoked anxiety attacks, by demonstrating that imipramine blocked panic attacks provoked by lactate in the laboratory.

The first direct comparison of an MAOI and a TCA as antipanic agents was undertaken in a placebo-controlled trial at Massachusetts General Hospital that demonstrated the two medications to be approximately equally effective (Sheehan et al. 1980). The psychopharmacological literature generated over the past three decades has been thoroughly reviewed, particularly by Ballenger (1986; Ballenger et al. 1977), Liebowitz (1986), and Fyer (1986).

It must be emphasized that the use of pharmacological treatments in general and benzodiazepines in particular for panic disorder represents a departure from the usual way in which anxiolytic pharmacotherapy has been prescribed. An analogy can be made with aspirin: Aspirin is often used for headache, in which case it is taken on an "as needed" basis in response to the immediate headache symptoms, usually only briefly, until the symptoms are resolved. This use is in contrast to the administration of aspirin for arthritis, for which the drug is recommended several times a day and over long periods, weeks or months, independent of the immediate level of symptoms. Thus, most anxiolytic and hypnotic benzodiazepines are used for acute stress reactions or short-term problems, akin to the model of aspirin use for headache. However, in the case of panic disorder, there is increasing use of benzodiazepines or antidepressants for long-term pharmacological treatment. These different uses are reflected in pharmacoepidemiological data, particularly studies by Balter (1984). (See Chapter 6.)

The hallmark of the pharmacological treatment of panic disorder is the blockade of panic attacks. The patient is first carefully told about the three features of the illness: panic attacks, anticipatory anxiety, and phobic avoidance. He or she is then reassured that, although panic attacks are extremely uncomfortable and psychologically disabling, they are not life threatening, do not cause psychosis, and do not provoke serious loss of control so as physically to endanger the patient or anyone else. Table 10 lists the various antipanic medications currently used, their usual dosage ranges, and their side effects. In general, the MAOIs are most commonly reserved for patients whose

Table 10.   Demonstrated effective drugs that block panic attacks

Generic name	Brand name	Dosage (mg/day)	Comment
Tricyclics			
Imipramine	Janimine SK-Pramine Tofranil	100–200[a]	
Desipramine	Norpramin	100–200[a]	Less anticholinergic than imipramine
Nortriptyline	Aventyl Pamelor	75–150	Possibly less orthostatic hypotension
MAOIs			
Phenelzine	Nardil	15–90	
Tranylcypromine	Parnate	10–30[b]	
Other agents			
Benzodiazepine			
Alprazolam	Xanax	1.0–4.0[c]	
Clonazepam	Klonopin	1.0–10	Not supported by controlled trials

Note.   MAOIs = monoamine oxidase inhibitors.
[a]Daily dose of 200–300 mg often needed to induce clinical remission.
[b]Daily dose up to 70 mg has been safely administered.
[c]Daily dose up to 6 mg may be required.

disorder is refractory to other medications. The clinician will choose between a TCA, such as imipramine, and alprazolam.

Monoamine Oxidase Inhibitors

Clinical experience with MAOIs in Great Britain has been responsible for a major part of the knowledge about the efficacy of that class of medication in panic disorder. Most recent studies have been on either phenelzine, the compound most widely studied and prescribed, or tranylcypromine; iproniazid, the compound initially studied, is no longer used. The early trials on MAOIs included patients with diagnoses of phobic anxiety and depersonalization syndrome.

In a landmark study by Sheehan and associates (1980) comparing MAOIs with TCAs, the diagnostic term "endogenous anxiety," roughly comparable to panic disorder, was used. Since the DSM-III-R (American Psychiatric Association 1987), almost all clinical studies with these compounds in this therapeutic area have been on panic disorder per se. Moderately high doses of phenelzine (45 mg to 90 mg per day) produced significant improvement in panic disorder symptoms and related anxiety symptoms in more than 75% of patients. The primary limitation in the use of MAOIs is the danger of hypertensive episodes if dietary restrictions are not followed. Also, the MAOIs have major interactions with many other drugs, including anesthetics, analgesics, other antidepressants, and anxiolytics, and potentiation with alcohol can occur. It is imperative, therefore, to monitor the ingestion of medication and foods by patients taking MAOIs. For these reasons, MAOIs are usually restricted to secondary use after initial failure with alprazolam, other benzodiazepines, or TCAs.

A patient with particularly refractory panic disorder may be an ideal candidate for treatment with an MAOI. Although phenelzine is most often prescribed, tranylcypromine has also been found effective. In several studies, MAOIs have been found to be marginally more effective than either alprazolam or imipramine.

Clinicians, especially in the United States, have shown some reluctance to prescribe MAOIs. Much of this fear comes from the need to place a patient on a tyramine-free diet to avoid hypertensive crises. Although the concern of clinicians is understandable, it must be emphasized that a tyramine-free diet is very easy to follow and that hypertensive crisis is rare in patients being treated with MAOIs. Phenelzine is usually initiated in a dose of 15 mg to 30 mg daily. Doses of less than 60 mg daily are rarely effective; up to 90 mg can be administered safely to most patients. As with TCAs, complete remission from panic attacks generally requires 4 to 12 weeks of treatment.

MAOIs induce substantial orthostatic hypotension in some patients, leading to postural dizziness and sometimes fatigue. Patients need to be told to rise slowly from a lying or sitting position, to increase salt and fluid intake, and occasionally to wear constrictive support hose. In some cases of severe postural hypotension, the addition of the mineralocorticoid fludrocortisone in doses of 0.1 mg two or three times daily for 2 weeks can stabilize blood pressure.

Additional side effects of MAOIs include weight gain, orgasmic dysfunction, peripheral edema, and hypomania. Although MAOIs are only weakly anticholinergic, some patients complain of dry mouth, constipation, and urinary retention. Tranylcypromine is especially likely to cause insomnia. Several MAOIs that exert reversible effects on monoamine oxidase and do not require dietary restrictions have been introduced in the past few years. The availability of these agents may well result in a substantial increase in MAOI use.

Tricyclic Antidepressants

General Considerations

TCAs are used in the specific treatment of panic disorder. Klein and Fink (1962) first showed that panic attacks can be blocked by the TCA imipramine. Acceptance of this now well-documented clinical effect was slow because, at the time, imipramine was believed to be an antidepressant exclusively. Unlike the benzodiazepines, administration of a single dose of imipramine did not lead to sedation, muscle relaxation, or an observable reduction in a patient's anxiety level. Nevertheless, the observation of Klein and Fink provided the basis for the theory that panic attacks are phenomenologically and biologically distinct from generalized anxiety. Generalized anxiety was originally thought to respond only to benzodiazepines and not to TCAs.

Imipramine

Approximately 12 placebo-controlled trials on panic disorder have been conducted with imipramine, all of which, except for a trial by Marks (1987), have demonstrated the superiority of imipramine over placebo (Lydiard and Ballenger 1987). However, after reanalysis of the Marks data, Raskin (1990) demonstrated a significant advantage of imipramine over placebo on most important outcome measures.

Imipramine, the prototype of the TCAs for the treatment of panic attacks, has important advantages and disadvantages. In the initial stages of administering imipramine, the drug sometimes causes a paradoxical increase in anxiety that usually resolves, after which other side effects more often associated with TCAs—dry mouth, constipation, orthostatic hypotension, difficulty urinating, and cycloplegia—often occur.

Imipramine rarely blocks panic attacks completely in fewer than 4 weeks. Once the medication becomes effective, however, it is generally well tolerated. The long half-life of imipramine allows the drug to be administered once daily, which usually is most conveniently done at bedtime. Withdrawal effects have not been reported during the slow tapering of imipramine in panic disorder patients. Panic attacks themselves do not generally reemerge immediately after the medication is stopped but, more frequently, recur weeks later in some patients.

If imipramine is chosen for the treatment of panic disorder, lower doses than those commonly used in treating depression are utilized in the initiation of treatment. One regimen is to begin with 10 mg at bedtime, increasing the dose by 10 mg every other day until a dose level of 50 mg is reached. This slow increase in dose usually obviates the paradoxical increase in anxiety that some patients experience. Panic blockade will be achieved in a minority of patients at doses as low as 50 mg per day. Hence, this dose should be maintained for several days. If, however, the dose is not effective by the end of this trial period, it is then increased by 25 mg every third day, up to 100 mg. If this dose regimen is not effective after 1 week, it is increased by 50 mg every third day. The average dose of imipramine that is effective in blocking panic attacks is approximately 200 mg daily. In some patients, doses up to 300 mg daily are needed and are generally well tolerated and safe. If patients are excessively bothered by anticholinergic side effects, a less anticholinergic TCA, such as desipramine, can be substituted. For patients who experience severe orthostatic hypotension, nortriptyline is often a successful substitute.

The dose of imipramine or desipramine required by patients with panic disorder ranges from 150 mg to as much as 300 mg. Response is generally seen after 8 to 12 weeks, with serum levels of TCAs at thresholds of 100 ng/ml to 150 ng/ml (Ballenger et al. 1984; Lydiard 1987; Mavissakalian and Jones 1990).

Clomipramine

Clomipramine, a derivative of the TCA class, was initially investigated as a treatment for major depression and more recently for obsessive-compulsive behavior. Because other TCAs, notably imipramine and desipramine, had been shown to be effective in the treatment of panic disorder, it seemed plausible that clomipramine would exert similar actions. In the 1970s, isolated reports of the favorable effects of clomipramine in the treatment of agoraphobia and social phobia were published (Beaumont 1977; Harding 1973; Waxman 1977). In these early reports, panic disorder was not specifically identified as a study diagnosis.

In 1980, Hoes and colleagues reported on a trial of six patients with hyperventilation syndrome who received clomipramine or imipramine and who appeared to have met the current criteria for panic disorder. Although the sample was small, the results were promising.

Gloger and others (1981) administered relatively low doses of clomipramine (often 50 mg per day or less) to 20 patients meeting DSM-III criteria for panic disorder or agoraphobia with panic attacks. Beneficial effects occurred within 10 to 14 days; after 8 weeks of treatment, 75% of the patients were asymptomatic. Since Gloger's study was published, a number of double-blind studies have been reported. Pecknold (1982) studied 24 patients with agoraphobia and 16 with social phobia. Panic attacks were noted in all the patients with agoraphobia and in 13 of 16 patients with social phobia. Pecknold administered a higher dose than previously used: up to 200 mg per day. The patients with agoraphobia seemed to improve more than those with social phobia.

Treatment with clomipramine is often accompanied by an early period of activation, with initial increases in anxiety lasting a few days to up to 5 to 10 days. Although this side effect can be managed with careful monitoring, reassurance, and dose reduction, it contributes to a relatively high patient dropout rate. However, in patients who completed 4 to 8 weeks of treatment, treatment resulted in a favorable response rate in the range of 70% to 75%.

Clomipramine has been investigated in open trials on the long-term treatment of panic disorder. Modigh and co-workers (1989) reported that, at 1- to 2-year follow-up after initiation of treatment with clomipramine, most patients were panic free, and the dose had been reduced to a range of 10 mg to 25 mg per day.

Adverse Effects of Tricyclic Antidepressants

Many patients experience difficulty with the autonomic and anticholinergic side effects of the TCAs. In the initial phase of treatment, more patients on TCAs are apt to leave a study because of adverse effects than those on alprazolam.

Some patients experience an activation phase, with insomnia, tremor, or both, during the first 2 weeks of treatment. This difficulty was particularly evident with TCAs that have a high affinity for serotonin receptors, such as clomipramine; it has also been reported in patients receiving the presynaptic serotonin reuptake blocking agent fluoxetine and traditional antidepressants, such as imipramine or, more frequently, desipramine (Pohl et al. 1988). However, if a patient can be sustained through this period (usually 10 to 14 days) with reassurance, dosage manipulation, and the use of adjunctive antianxiety agents, efficacy comparable to that of alprazolam will be exhibited within 4 to 8 weeks.

With TCAs, anticholinergic effects occur such as dry mouth, constipation, difficulty attaining orgasm, and other atropine-like complications. Weight gain can be as much as 1 pound per month. Approximately 25% of patients experience weight gain of 20 pounds or more (Noyes et al. 1989b). Finally, the TCAs have a limited safety margin in overdose, which may pose a problem if a patient is suicidal.

Taylor and associates (1990) have been investigating the cardiovascular and metabolic effects of long-term medication with TCAs and have raised the issue of the possible association of long-term imipramine treatment with increased cardiovascular risk. Although much information about the cardiovascular side effects of TCAs is available, they are generally safe in a clinically healthy population, particularly a young adult population such as that afflicted by panic disorder. Orthostatic hypotension, the major cardiovascular side effect, is dangerous primarily in elderly patients in whom autonomic control of peripheral vascular tone has deteriorated and who are at substantial risk of serious injury from a fall. In such patients, nortriptyline may be a better choice than imipramine because nortriptyline has been shown to induce less orthostatic hypotension. In any event, if a TCA is used in an elderly person, blood pressure should be carefully monitored.

TCAs increase cardiac conduction times through the atrioventricular node, thus prolonging PR and QRS intervals in most patients.

Again, in clinically healthy patients, electrocardiographic (ECG) changes are generally insignificant. In patients older than 50 years, an ECG should be obtained before the patient begins taking a TCA.

Clinical Issues

It is best to begin treatment with TCAs, including imipramine, and clomipramine at a relatively low dose (i.e., 10 mg per day). A substantial minority of patients will experience stimulation-like effects. Gradual increases of the dose over several weeks improves patient compliance and results in a higher percentage of patients who are able to tolerate therapeutic drug levels. Many experts emphasize titrating doses of TCAs to more than 150 mg per day.

Dose During Long-Term Treatment

During the recommended initial period of treatment (i.e., the first 6 months), the patient should be maintained on the highest dose of imipramine tolerable. That is, if the patient has responded to a dose of 200 mg daily, this dose should be maintained for the entire 6 months unless supervening side effects mandate reduction. The question whether there is a specific maintenance dose of imipramine for treating panic disorder has not been determined, although it seems clear that maintance doses of TCAs or alprazolam can be significantly lower than initial doses. Once panic attacks are blocked, panic disorder may improve spontaneously. Older benzodiazepines, such as diazepam and lorazepam, can be administered concomitantly with a TCA to manage anticipatory anxiety until the full antipanic effect of the TCA is attained. Phobic avoidance usually decreases markedly when panic attacks are blocked, but desensitization treatment is required occasionally to fully relieve phobic avoidance.

No study to date has systematically addressed the length of time required to adequately treat panic disorder. In clinical practice, an attempt to discontinue the medication should be made 6 to 13 months after clinical remission from panic attacks. Imipramine can generally be tapered over a period of 2 weeks without encountering the flu-like symptoms that commonly follow abrupt discontinuation. However, tapering should be even slower, with careful observation of the patient for relapse of panic attacks. It has been reported that up to 80% of panic disorder patients will remain in remission after a 6-month course of imipramine. Rates of relapse, however, have been scientifically studied in only a few trials (Zitrin et al. 1983). Some studies suggest that relapse rates are much higher (e.g., Versiani et al. 1985); some patients apparently require much longer drug treatment.

Benzodiazepines

General Considerations

The first benzodiazepine, synthesized in 1957, was chlordiazepoxide. Other benzodiazepines that are currently available in the United States include diazepam, oxazepam, clorazepate, lorazepam, prazepam, flurazepam, halazepam, temazepam, alprazolam, triazolam, and—as an anticonvulsant—clonazepam (see Table 11 for their half-lives and the daily doses given for approved indications). Some other benzodiazepines that are available in international markets are undergoing study in the United States. All the benzodiazepines have roughly similar anxiolytic, sedative-hypnotic, and anticonvulsive properties, although they are promoted for various indications. Mod-

Table 11. Benzodiazepine drugs used in treatment of anxiety

Generic name	Brand name	Half-life (hour)	Dosage (mg/day)
Long-acting			
Diazepam	Valium	60	2–60
Chlordiazepoxide	Librium	24–48	15–100
Clorazepate	Tranxene	100	7.5–60
Halazepam	Paxipam	50	60–160
Prazepam	Centrax	100	20–60
Clonazepam[a]	Klonopin	34	1.5–20
Flurazepam[b]	Dalmane	100	15–30
Short-acting			
Oxazepam	Serax	8	30–120
Lorazepam	Ativan	15	2–6
Alprazolam[b]	Xanax	12	0.5–6
Temazepam[c]	Restoril	11	15–30
Triazolam[b, c]	Halcion	2	0.125–0.5
Midazolam[d]	Versed	2	2–4

[a] Marketed as an anticonvulsant.
[b] Marketed as a hypnotic.
[c] Triazolobenzodiazepine.
[d] Only manufactured in parenteral form.

est pharmacodynamic differences, as well as important pharmaco-kinetic differences, may play a role in differentiating the various benzodiazepines.

The concept that anxiety disorders are distinct clinical entities did not gain widespread acceptance until the 1980s because of differential drug responses. Before publication of the DSM-III, anxiety was gener-ally considered a symptom associated with the stress of everyday life and with many medical and psychiatric illnesses. One class of drug—the benzodiazepines—has been virtually synonymous with antianxi-ety drugs since its introduction in the 1960s. These medications, which replaced meprobamate and barbiturates for almost all patients, were found to effectively reduce anxiety levels with minimal side ef-fects. At the same time that the benzodiazepines were introduced, however, researchers began accumulating evidence that anxiety was not an amorphous or homogeneous symptom but rather a generic clas-sification for several specific syndromes.

Through the 1960s and 1970s, the conventional wisdom was that standard benzodiazepines, including diazepam and chlordiazepoxide, were ineffective in blocking panic disorder. This point of view was ex-pressed by Zitrin and associates (1980, 1983), Sheehan (1982), and others. Although benzodiazepines were widely used in the treatment of what today is called panic disorder, this practice was not supported by any systematic trials or the experience of psychopharmacologists.

A development emerged during 1980 to 1982 with observations in uncontrolled studies of the ability of alprazolam to block panic attacks. These observations were reported in Canada by Chouinard and asso-ciates (1982) and in the United States by Sheehan (1982) and Alexan-der and Alexander (1986). The doses used, 4 mg to 6 mg per day, were considerably higher than those normally used for anxiety. Gradually, a small number of controlled studies confirmed this observation and prompted the Upjohn Company to initiate the Cross-National Collab-orative Panic Study (CNCPS) to test out the efficacy of alprazolam for panic disorder (Klerman 1988; Klerman et al. 1986).

Confirmatory data on the long-term treatment of panic disorder, obtained by direct observation, began to appear in the 1970s. In an open study, Gross (1977) treated patients with "anxiety neurosis" or "depressive neurosis" for 6 months; mood ratings were obtained at 1, 3, and 6 months. Thirty-four patients received lorazepam, 3 mg to 6 mg per day, and 16 received diazepam at comparable doses. Improve-ment was maintained to the end of the study. In a similar study with "psychoneurotic patients with severe manifest anxiety," Fabre and colleagues (1981) found sustained improvement without dose escalation over a 6-month period in 63 patients taking alprazolam and 32 taking diazepam. In a placebo-controlled study with "chronically anxious outpatients," Rickels and others (1983) found improvement sustained to 22 weeks with diazepam. Cohn and Wilcox (1984) made similar observations in a study of patients with "moderate to moderately severe anxiety" treated with alprazolam or lorazepam over 16 weeks. Rickels and associates (1988) found sustained effectiveness of chlorazepate over 6 months in patients with generalized anxiety disorder or panic disorder. In several series of case reports of patients with panic disorder treated with clonazepam, improvement without dose escalation was maintained for observation periods up to 68 weeks (Herman et al. 1987; Spier et al. 1986; Tesar and Rosenbaum 1986).

Alprazolam

Alprazolam has the largest empirical data base because of the multicenter CNCPS. The CNCPS was conducted in two phases. Phase I compared alprazolam with placebo at eight sites (five in the United States, two in Canada, and one in Australia). The results of the study demonstrated that patients with panic disorder who were treated with alprazolam experienced significant reductions in the number and intensity of panic attacks in avoidance behavior and in fear, often in the first and second weeks. After completion of the 8-week research protocol in Phase I of the CNCPS, 69 of the panic disorder patients continued taking alprazolam and 16 continued taking placebo for an additional 6 months (Ballenger et al. 1988). Of patients receiving alprazolam, 70% experienced no panic attacks by the end of 8 months. None of the patients acquired a tolerance. The mean dose decreased from 5.7 ± 2.2 mg per day to 4.7 ± 2.1 mg per day. Most patients continued to improve in social functioning and reduced their phobic avoidance behavior (Dupont et al. 1992).

On the basis of the findings from Phase I, the Phase II comparative study, which compared alprazolam with the standard antipanic compound imipramine and with placebo at 12 sites in North and South America and western Europe, was started. After 8 weeks of treatment, the two active drugs were more effective than placebo on most outcome measures, including panic attacks, anticipatory episodes, and overall phobia.

After completion of the 8-week research protocol in Phase II of the

CNCPS, patients from 4 of the 12 study sites who had improved were continued on the same double-blind treatment they had been receiving for up to 6 additional months. Of the patients entering the long-term treatment study from the selected study sites, 78 (58%) patients were taking alprazolam, 65 (49%) were taking imipramine, and 38 (27%) were taking placebo (Curtis et al. 1990). All three groups had improved during the 8-week study (active treatments more than placebo and about equal to each other). Patients were seen monthly during the extension naturalistic study. Clinical assessments, ratings, and dose adjustments under double-blind conditions were conducted as they had been during the acute study.

All three groups maintained or extended their improvement over the 6 additional months without any significant change in dose (see Figures 1 and 2). More than twice as many alprazolam- and imipramine-treated patients than placebo-treated patients remained in treatment for the full 8 months. The patients who received active medications had slightly better scores on symptom measures than did the placebo patients who remained in the study. It is not clear whether the dropouts represent failure to sustain improvement, relapse, side effects, or other phenomena. Although dropout rates somewhat obscure

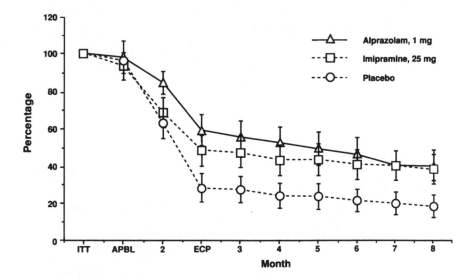

Figure 1. Retention in study with 95% confidence intervals. ITT = intent to treat; APBL = acute phase baseline; month 2 = end of acute phase; ECP = enter chronic phase.

the findings in this study, the accumulated evidence clearly shows that long-term treatment of panic disorder with benzodiazepines is feasible and results in sustained clinical improvement.

Additionally, Schweitzer and co-workers (1993) reported a prospective placebo-controlled comparison of alprazolam and imipramine in 107 patients treated for 8 months. Most patients who continued taking medication for the 8-month period were free of panic by the end of treatment. The dose of alprazolam was 5.7 mg per day, which was well tolerated. The dose of imipramine of 175 mg per day was associated with less improvement and higher attrition.

The efficacy demonstrated by alprazolam in the treatment of panic disorder raised the question of whether alprazolam might be different from other benzodiazepines. Two explanations, pharmacodynamic and pharmacokinetic, were offered. The pharmacodynamic explanation emphasized findings showing the effects of alprazolam on downregulation of beta receptors (Sethy and Hodges 1982) and suggested a common mode of action for antipanic and antidepressant effects. Laboratory studies also indicated that alprazolam reduced the firing rate of the locus ceruleus, the central neural adrenergic center, in ways similar to the effects of imipramine and the MAOIs.

The pharmacokinetic explanation emphasized the high affinity of alprazolam for the benzodiazepine and gamma-aminobutyric acid

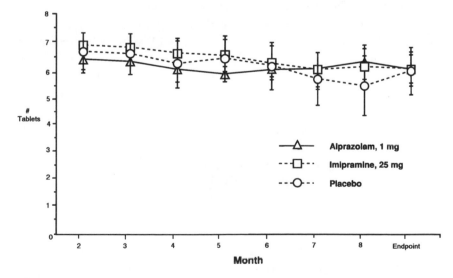

Figure 2. Average number of tablets per day with 95% confidence intervals.

(GABA) receptor complex and the low-dose formulation. Later studies compared lorazepam with alprazolam (Charney and Woods 1989) and compared alprazolam with diazepam (R. Noyes, G. Burrows, unpublished data, 1988). It appears that if a dose of diazepam were raised high enough (a dose ratio of 10 mg of diazepam to 1 mg of alprazolam), panic attacks would be blocked; 10 mg of diazepam appears to be equiactive to 1 mg of alprazolam in blocking panic. Therefore, 50 mg of diazepam is roughly equivalent to 5 mg of alprazolam in antipanic activity. However, considerably more sedation occurs with this dose of diazepam than with the equivalent dose of alprazolam. Clinical experience suggests that the clinical superiority of alprazolam is largely attributed to the wide margin between doses that provide clinical efficacy and those that produce sedative adverse effects.

Other Benzodiazepines

The use of other benzodiazepines, notably clonazepam, for panic disorder is under investigation (Katon 1990; Rosenbaum 1987). In one double-blind comparison, clonazepam was roughly comparable in efficacy to alprazolam (Beaudry et al. 1985). Table 11 lists other benzodiazepines used to treat panic disorder.

Adverse Effects

Patients taking benzodiazepines sometimes experience early sedation, but that effect resolves rapidly, particularly when it is managed with dosage titration. Sexual side effects have also been reported. When benzodiazepines are discontinued, withdrawal symptoms, rebound symptoms, or both occur in some patients, especially if the dose was tapered rapidly. Occasionally, the benzodiazepines, including alprazolam, evoke various disinhibition (release) phenomena that may be based on specific types of character pathology and that may jeopardize the treatment process and interfere with the patient's interpersonal, occupational, and marital-family functioning. When benzodiazepines are taken for long periods, they may produce ataxia and cognitive impairment, particularly in the elderly. Long duration of treatment can increase the risks of withdrawal on discontinuation.

Abuse Potential

Concern has been expressed about the possible abuse potential of benzodiazepines in the treatment of panic disorder. Abuse potential refers to the capacity of a drug to induce effects perceived by the subject as pleasurable and that result in behaviors to repeat the experience, including obtaining sources of supply and repeated self-administration. Addictive potential refers to drug-seeking behavior despite social and legal contraindications, a loss of control with occasional use, and the prominence of drug use in the psychological life and behavior of a person. Griffiths and Roache (1985) and Lader (1992) reviewed the general concern about the abuse potential of the benzodiazepines. They emphasized differences in response between nonalcoholic persons and persons with a history of alcoholism, other substance abuse, or both in rank ordering of drug preference between nonalcoholic individuals and individuals with a history of alcoholism, other substance abuse, or both. Whereas nonalcoholic persons prefer placebos to benzodiazepines or fail to discriminate between placebos and benzodiazepines, those with a history of substance abuse report more euphoric effect from a standard dose of a benzodiazepine than control subjects. Patients with a history of substance abuse also prefer amphetamines and barbiturates to placebo. The pharmacological basis for the difference between nonalcoholic persons and persons with substance abuse problems has not been established.

Effect of Comorbidity With Substance Abuse

In persons who abuse alcohol or drugs, benzodiazepines tend to be secondary drugs of abuse taken to enhance intoxication effects of another drug, often in a quasi-therapeutic manner, for sleep induction, reduction of anxiety associated with drug dependence, treatment of unwanted withdrawal symptoms from another dependence-producing drug, or a combination of those actions. Thus, there is a high likelihood of finding people who abuse alcohol in populations experiencing discontinuation symptoms and increased benzodiazepine abuse among alcoholic persons. Benzodiazepines may be cross-tolerant to alcohol and may be used in treating alcohol withdrawal symptoms. This finding suggests that benzodiazepines are contraindicated in patients with panic disorder and comorbid substance abuse.

Dependence

Physical dependence has been defined in many ways. In the studies described in this review, it is defined as a physiological and biochemical change in the central neural adrenergic center produced by the chronic administration of a drug such that cessation of drug intake or rapid reduction of dosage is followed by the appearance of a characteristic withdrawal syndrome or abstinence syndrome. Currently, there is no physiological or biochemical test to directly determine whether physical dependence has occurred in a person. The occurrence of the state of physical dependence is inferred in humans from animal studies and from the occurrence of withdrawal reactions on discontinuation of medication. Thus, a firm diagnosis of physical dependence cannot be made on the basis of a medical history or an examination without evidence of a withdrawal reaction to dose reduction or drug cessation.

Clinical Discontinuation Reactions

It is now widely accepted that a range of patient reactions will occur after a reduction in alprazolam dose. There are four types of outcomes: 1) absence of reactions, 2) withdrawal, 3) rebound, and 4) relapse. However, in clinical samples, withdrawal, rebound, and relapse often occur simultaneously; therefore, their differentiation is often difficult in practice. A large percentage of patients, which varies from study to study, will not experience a discontinuation reaction (i.e., they will be able to discontinue alprazolam without adverse effect or subjective discomfort). The available data indicate that 20% to 80% of patients do not experience discontinuation reactions, but most of the more recent studies place this rate at 35% to 45% (Ballenger 1991). A major determinant of the frequency of no reaction is the rate of dose taper, but other factors may be involved.

Withdrawal reactions represent the physical manifestations of the dependence potential of the benzodiazepines. The central characteristics of benzodiazepine withdrawal reaction are shown in Table 12. Pecknold and colleagues (1988), among others, concluded that there is a characteristic symptom profile of benzodiazepine withdrawal. However, in addition to the symptoms in Table 12, withdrawal-type reactions may be accompanied by various types of nonspecific depressive, anxiety, and tension symptoms, which makes differential diagnosis between benzodiazepine withdrawal and relapse clinically difficult.

The temporal sequence of reactions provides one means to make a differential diagnosis. Withdrawal reactions of short-acting benzodiazepines, such as alprazolam, tend to occur relatively early, whereas withdrawal associated with medium- and longer acting benzodiazepines, notably diazepam, may be more gradual in onset and perhaps less severe. Symptoms present 3 weeks after discontinuation, however, can be considered relapse (Ballenger 1991).

Table 12.   Benzodiazepine withdrawal syndrome symptoms

Newly emergent; not part of anxiety disorder

- ▼ Confusion
- ▼ Diarrhea
- ▼ Clouded sensorium
- ▼ Blurred vision
- ▼ Heightened sensory perception

- ▼ Muscle cramps
- ▼ Dysosmia
- ▼ Muscle twitches
- ▼ Paresthesia
- ▼ Decreased appetite
- ▼ Weight loss

Note. If treatment is stopped abruptly, possible convulsion and delirium may result.
Source. Pecknold et al. 1988, used with permission.

Rebound

A moderate percentage of patients (10% to 35%) will experience rebound when they rapidly discontinue benzodiazepines (Pecknold et al. 1988). Rebound represents the temporary return of anxiety symptoms to a level greater than that experienced by a patient when he or she first entered the study. Rebound, which includes significant electroencephalographic (EEG) changes, was first noted with hypnotic benzodiazepines. For anxiolytic agents, rebound entails the return of anxiety symptoms, panic attacks in particular. In a comparison between alprazolam and diazepam, Noyes and associates (1991) reported a rebound in the number of panic attacks occurring during the second or third day, which receded rapidly thereafter.

Relapse refers to the return of the original anxiety disorder for which the patient sought treatment and for the most part is reduced in severity and frequency after short-term treatment. Relapse rates vary from study to study (Table 13).

Factors Influencing Benzodiazepine Withdrawal in Panic Disorder Patients

As shown in Table 14, several factors have been identified and hypothesized to influence the frequency, intensity, and duration of the benzodiazepine withdrawal syndrome. Most of the factors are common in all clinical syndromes for which benzodiazepines are indicated, but some are reported to be more applicable to patients with panic disorder. Some of the factors are discussed next.

Pharmacological properties.   Much attention is given to the pharmacological properties of a drug, including its half-life. Short-acting drugs are believed to be more likely to induce withdrawal reactions than benzodiazepines with long half-lives.

Social environment and psychological history.   Factors affecting benzodiazepine withdrawal symptoms in panic disorder patients include a history of alcohol abuse, drug abuse, or both; personality traits, including neuroticism, impulsivity, and passivity; interpersonal mistrust and a strong need for control; social attitudes about use of benzodiazepine; the information a patient has about the manifestations of withdrawal; and the degrees of moral criticism and social approval by members of the patient's family, friends, and colleagues.

Patient diagnosis.   There is some suggestion that patients with panic disorder may be more susceptible to withdrawal symptoms because of a greater sensitivity of neural adrenergic receptors.

Clinical treatment decisions.   Higher dosage, longer duration, and abrupt or rapid dose taper have been implicated in increases in the frequency and intensity of withdrawal reactions.

Adjunctive treatment.   Attempts to treat benzodiazepine withdrawal with use of medication have been undertaken in a number of

Table 13.   Relapse studies

Study	Initial treatment	Length of follow-up (years)	Relapse (%)
Kelly et al. 1970	1 year MAOI	1 year	50
Zitrin et al. 1983	6 months IMI[a]	1 year	19–31
Sheehan 1986	8 months IMI/MAOI/ALP	1 year	70–90
Mavissakalian and Michelson 1986b	3 months IMI[a]	2 years	28
Zitrin 1987	6 months IMI[a]	5 years	17

Note.   MAOI = monoamine oxidase inhibitor; IMI = imipramine; ALP = alprazolam.
[a] Combined behavior therapy.
Source.   Roy-Byrne and Lydiard 1989.

studies. The most notable recent studies have assessed carbamazepine for this use, but only limited success has been reported (Rickels et al. 1991).

Current management of withdrawal entails a gradual dose taper during medication discontinuation as well as patient and family education, reassurance, and support.

Serotonin Reuptake Blocking Agents

The utility of selective serotonin reuptake inhibitors (SSRIs) for the treatment of panic disorder was suggested by two findings: 1) the implication of the serotonergic neurotransmitter system in the pathogenesis of panic disorder (see Chapter 3 for additional relevant information) and 2) the antipanic effect of older antidepressants that nonselectively block serotonin reuptake, such as clomipramine (see the subsection of this chapter). Before the SSRI zimelidine was withdrawn from the market in the United Kingdom because of rare but serious adverse effects (e.g., Guillain-Barré syndrome), it was compared with imipramine and placebo in a 6-week double-blind study of 44 patients with agoraphobia and panic attacks (Evans et al. 1986). Zimelidine was more effective than imipramine, as well as placebo, in reducing the number of panic attacks.

Fluvoxamine is the best studied SSRI in panic disorder. In a double-blind study comparing fluvoxamine with clomipramine in 50 patients for 6 weeks (Den Boer et al. 1987), fluvoxamine was found to be equally as efficacious as clomipramine in reducing the frequency of

---

Table 14.   Benzodiazepine withdrawal syndrome—factors influencing frequency, intensity, and duration

Pharmacologic	**Patient diagnosis**
Half-life of drug	**Clinical**
Receptor affinity	Dose
Potency	Duration
Patient	Taper schedule
Alcohol and/or drug abuse	
Personality: neuroticism,	
impulsivity, passivity	
Attitudes toward benzodiazepines	

panic attacks and phobic avoidance. In a double-blind, 6-week study of fluvoxamine versus maprotiline in 44 patients (Den Boer and Westenberg 1988), fluvoxamine was superior to maprotiline, an effective TCA that selectively inhibits norepinephrine uptake, in the reduction of panic attacks and avoidance behavior. This finding suggested that the mechanism responsible for the antipanic activity of antidepressants in panic disorder is not the same as that responsible for antidepressant activity. In a third double-blind study (Den Boer and Westenberg 1990a), fluvoxamine was compared with ritanserin, a specific 5-HT$_2$ (5-hydroxytryptamine [serotonin]) antagonist, and placebo in 60 patients with panic disorder. After 8 weeks of treatment, the number of panic attacks was markedly lower in patients who were treated with fluvoxamine compared with those who had received placebo; the fluvoxamine-treated patients also experienced a subsequent decrease in avoidance behavior. Ritanserin was found to be ineffective.

In a dose-ranging study of 50 mg, 100 mg, and 150 mg of fluvoxamine (J. A. Den Boer, unpublished data, 1992), the three doses were about equally efficacious. However, the incidence of side effects was lowest in patients who received the 50-mg dose (although side effects were minor for all patients), suggesting that low doses of fluvoxamine may be effective for the treatment of panic disorder.

There have been a limited number of reports of the use of fluoxetine in panic disorder. In an open study of 25 panic disorder patients with or without agoraphobia, Schneier and colleagues (1990) found that fluoxetine given for 12 months produced moderate to marked improvement in 19 patients (76%). Four patients (16%) discontinued fluoxetine because of adverse effects. L. Solyom and co-workers (1991) reported that two patients with panic disorder, agoraphobia, and depression who received fluoxetine, 80 mg per day, each experienced an amelioration of panic disorder without concomitant weight gain. Other SSRIs, such as sertraline and paroxetine, seem promising as antipanic agents from a theoretical perspective, but supportive data have not yet been generated.

The mechanism of action of the antipanic effect of SSRIs appears to be related to the serotonergic system but requires further characterization. When fluvoxamine has been used to treat panic disorder, patients have typically experienced a temporary (during the first 2 weeks of treatment) worsening of anxiety symptoms before improvement has occurred. It has been hypothesized (Den Boer and Westenberg 1990b) that treatment with a serotonin reuptake inhibitor initially stimulates 5-HT receptors and subsequently downregulates 5-HT$_2$ receptors, which results in an amelioration of the clinical condition. In the aforementioned study of fluvoxamine versus ritanserin, the lack of efficacy of ritanserin suggested that the 5-HT$_2$ receptor subtype may not play a role in panic disorder. 5-HT receptor subtypes that may be responsible for the efficacy of SSRIs in panic disorder, particularly the 5-HT$_{1A}$ receptor, remain under investigation.

Depression and Psychopharmacological Treatment Response

High rates of comorbidity between panic disorder and depression have been reported in a number of epidemiological and clinical studies (see Chapter 2; for an overview, see Maser and Cloninger 1990). Comorbidity may affect the response of panic disorder to medication.

Marks suggested that the therapeutic effects of antidepressants in panic disorder are not due to an intrinsic antipanic or antiphobic activity but rather to a general effect on affect, particularly on depression (Marks et al. 1983). He arrived at this conclusion because his sample of phobic patients, which was unusual in that they did not respond to imipramine, had been selected for their low severity of depression. However, he did not perform an internal analysis comparing outcomes among his patients who were relatively more depressed at baseline with those who were less depressed. This issue was already addressed in the 1970s by others. Kelly and colleagues (1970), in a retrospective chart study, found that initial depression did not influence the degree of improvement in anxiety symptoms treated with MAOIs. Tyrer and associates (1973) conducted a small, controlled study of phenelzine and placebo that showed no relation between initial depression and the relief of phobic symptoms.

A series of larger controlled studies consistently confirmed these early findings (Mavissakalian 1987; McNair and Kahn 1981; Sheehan et al. 1980; Zitrin et al. 1980, 1983). All these investigators carried out analyses within their samples specifically to examine the association between initial depression and the response of panic and agoraphobia to antidepressant treatment. Zitrin and colleagues (1983) found a modest negative correlation between initial depression and response to medication among both imipramine- and placebo-treated patients.

These issues were most recently examined using data from Phase I and Phase II of the CNCPS. Klerman (1990) reported no difference in the antipanic response between depressed patients and those who were not depressed. (Patients with serious depressive conditions were excluded.) Moreover, there were relatively few differences between the response to imipramine and the response to alprazolam. Contrary to expectation, imipramine was not more effective than alprazolam for the relief of depressive symptoms. However, the evidence at present seems to favor the view that depression, as it is commonly found in patients with panic disorder, is not a major determinant of the response to treatment with either antidepressants or alprazolam.

Comparative Psychopharmacological Studies

Until the early 1980s, few trials had directly compared the antidepressant classes with each other or with the benzodiazepines. Subsequently, Versiani and associates (1985) reported a large, uncontrolled trial comparing clomipramine, alprazolam, and tranylcypromine, finding similar, excellent results with the three medications. Ballenger and colleagues (1987) compared imipramine, alprazolam, phenelzine, and lorazepam in a 12-week open trial, finding the efficacies of those medications roughly equivalent. Uhlenhuth and associates (1989) reported a fixed-dose, double-blind comparison of alprazolam and imipramine in panic disorder patients. Although more patients taking imipramine than those taking alprazolam dropped out during the first 2 weeks of treatment (probably because of adverse effects), those remaining in the trial responded at least as well to imipramine as to alprazolam.

However, the recent CNCPS trial, with its careful methodology and large patient samples, provided a definitive, placebo-controlled comparison between imipramine and alprazolam. After 8 weeks of treatment, the two active drugs were more effective than placebo on nearly all clinical outcome measures, but they did not differ significantly from each other (de la Fuente 1988). Table 15 summarizes the advantages and disadvantages of the various types of antipanic drugs (Ballenger 1990).

Long-Term Psychopharmacological Treatment of Panic Disorder

The research on the treatment of panic disorder was dominated in the early 1970s and 1980s by the need to evaluate the role of various psy-

chopharmacological agents alone and in comparison with psychological treatment for short-term treatment (4 to 12 weeks). Out of this
research emerged wide agreement on the efficacy of drug treatment
for panic disorder with members of three classes of compounds. Moreover, the U.S. Food and Drug Administration (FDA) approved alprazolam for the treatment of panic disorder in 1990. This approval
represents the first time the FDA has approved a compound for panic
disorder.

In the late 1980s attention became increasingly focused on long-
term treatment of panic disorder (more than 6 months). Reports of the
high relapse rates (Versiani et al. 1985) after discontinuation from
short-term treatment led many clinicians to prescribe continued medication for their patients. Therefore, considerable clinical experience
has been generated with long-term treatment with TCAs (Noyes et al.
1989b). Researchers have become increasingly aware of the similari-

Table 15.   Advantages and disadvantages of various drugs as antipanic
agents

Drug	Advantages	Disadvantages
Monoamine oxidase inhibitors	Better antiphobic Antidepressant	Dietary restrictions Delayed onset Insomnia Orthostatic hypotension Weight gain Sexual effects Mania (bipolar patients)
Tricyclic antidepressants	Single daily dose Antidepressant Well-studied Some generics available	Delayed onset Activation symptoms Anticholinergic Orthostatic hypotension Sexual effects Mania (bipolar patients) Weight gain
Benzodiazepines	Rapid onset Well-tolerated Reduces anticipatory anxiety	Sedation Multiple dosing Dependence/withdrawal

Source. Ballenger 1990.

ties between the treatment of panic disorder and the treatment of major depression with antidepressant drugs (Hirschfeld 1990; Klerman 1990; Kupfer 1991). Gradually, a small body of literature has emerged on the safety and efficacy of long-term treatment, addressing, for example, dosage, duration of treatment, placebo effect, role of psychological treatment, and problems of discontinuation.

In the late 1980s and now in the 1990s, attention has shifted from concern over the management of short-term pharmacological treatment to long-term treatment. Clinicians have become increasingly aware of the necessity for long-term treatment for a large proportion of patients with panic disorder. However, the optimal duration of treatment has not been defined, and the long-term use of all available antipanic agents is associated with some problems. Continued use of both TCAs and MAOIs is associated with weight gain. MAOIs can also produce hypertensive crises and hyperpyrexic reactions. Benzodiazepines taken for long periods may produce ataxia and cognitive impairment and are associated with high risks of dependence and withdrawal.

Despite these problems, long-term treatment of panic disorder (6 or 12 months or more) has found favor because continued treatment helps in consolidating gains and overcoming social isolation and avoidant behavior (Schatzberg and Ballenger 1991). Early discontinuation of medication has been associated with high rates of relapse (Fyer et al. 1987b).

Tricyclic Antidepressants in Long-Term Treatment

The efficacy of long-term treatment with TCAs, usually imipramine, has been described in a small number of uncontrolled studies conducted in the United States (Noyes et al. 1989b). Curtis and colleagues (1990) reviewed data from the CNCPS that showed that 6 additional months of treatment with alprazolam or imipramine extended the results beyond the initial months of short-term treatment. Clinical improvement was maintained, and there was no dose escalation. There is a large body of experience with adverse effects associated with the long-term use of TCAs in affective disorders, in particular, recurrent unipolar depression. This experience is likely to be similar in patients with panic disorder (Noyes et al. 1989b). Distressing effects may emerge on the sudden discontinuation of TCAs. Such effects have included rebound, hypomanic episodes, and sleep disturbance. The effects have not been interpreted as physical dependence or withdrawal reactions but as rebound anticholinergic sensitivity.

Alprazolam and Other Benzodiazepines

Whereas tolerance occurs rapidly to the sedative-hypnotic effects of alprazolam, tolerance does not develop to its antipanic and other therapeutic effects. Dose escalation did not occur in the few studies that have been conducted on long-term treatment with alprazolam; instead, there were reductions in dose over time (Burrows 1990a, 1990b; Dupont et al. 1992; Nagy et al. 1989). Uncontrolled studies of long-term treatment in open trials have been reported by Nagy and colleagues (1989). Adverse effects are relatively uncommon during long-term treatment. Tolerance to the sedative effects usually occurs during the first weeks of treatment; subsequently, patients are seldom bothered by drowsiness or lethargy. With data from the CNCPS Phase I, Dupont and colleagues (1992) reported patient reactions to discontinuation after long-term treatment that included both withdrawal reactions and relapse. They also described a group of patients who were reluctant to discontinue the medication, fearing that their panic disorder and other symptoms of anxiety would return. The crucial determinants in the clinical management of long-term treatment seem to be the attitudes of the patient and the physician and the rate of taper (Pecknold 1990). Many patients and their physicians mistake relapse symptoms as benzodiazepine withdrawal symptoms and stop treatment prematurely. Others make the opposite error, mistaking benzodiazepine withdrawal as evidence of relapse, and continue treatment unnecessarily while increasing the risk of dependency. Careful clinical assessment of the time course of symptoms usually distinguishes withdrawal from relapse.

Another question about the maintenance treatment of panic disorder pertains to differences in the long-term benefits and risks of various classes of drugs. Available data indicate that the therapeutic effects of alprazolam and imipramine can be maintained up to 8 months. However, rebound and withdrawal appear to be more frequent after discontinuing alprazolam, especially when it is discontinued relatively rapidly (Pecknold 1990; Pecknold et al. 1988). It is suspected, although not proven, that rebound provokes relapse and ultimately prompts a return to medication. In that case, relapse might be expected to be more frequent after stopping a benzodiazepine, which is associated with rebound more frequently than an antidepressant; there is preliminary evidence that relapse occurs more frequently with benzodiazepines than with TCAs.

Patients who have been free of panic attacks and have done well in general with imipramine for 6 to 12 months should be advised to discontinue the drug gradually (e.g., to make a reduction of 25 mg in the daily dose every month), the final goal being to discontinue the drug completely. If symptoms return, consideration should be given to restarting the drug, a measure that is almost always effective. In that event, however, the risks and benefits of continued administration must be weighed. Potentially serious adverse effects include successful suicide attempts using the drugs, sometimes fatal hypertensive crises, febrile reactions with MAOIs, and seizures. Orthostatic hypotension, leading to falls, and cardiac arrhythmias are more apt to occur in medically ill or elderly patients. Weight gain is a frequent long-term consequence, and changes in heart rate and blood pressure with TCAs carry a potential for adversely affecting health over the long term. Many of these risks, although relatively low, increase with duration of administration.

Before any attempt to discontinue medication, patients should be advised to reduce the dose gradually to half of the original dose. If a return of symptoms is experienced, the dose should be restored to the lowest effective level and kept at that level for another 6 months to a year, at which time the next attempt to discontinue the drug can be made. If a TCA is stopped abruptly, anticholinergic withdrawal symptoms, including nausea, tremor, headache, and insomnia, may begin in 24 hours; with a gradual decrease in dose, these symptoms are less likely to occur. Rebound anxiety and other withdrawal symptoms may occur after discontinuation of TCAs or MAOIs, but the frequency of such phenomena is not known. Patients who are successful in discontinuing a drug should not reinstitute it unless or until symptoms of the original disorder recur.

If two or three attempts to discontinue an antidepressant prove unsuccessful, a patient probably should continue taking the drug indefinitely. Patients often are disappointed when symptoms reappear and view their reappearance as a personal failure or a failure of the medication. However, patients are often better able to accept long-term maintenance therapy after two or three attempts at discontinuation have failed. A few patients find that there are periods when they need antidepressant medication and other periods when they remain well without it. Usually, a gradual reduction in dose will result in a smaller need for a drug, but occasionally a patient will recognize a pattern of changing symptoms that serves as an indication that medication is again required. In such cases, maintaining the lowest dose possible for controlling symptoms may be the best treatment alternative.

Psychological Treatments

General Considerations

In the mid-1980s, cognitive-behavioral therapists began to develop treatment methods for panic anxiety without agoraphobic avoidance. Some therapists regarded panic attacks as different from other forms of anxiety only quantitatively and used therapies utilized for other types of anxiety disorder, such as relaxation and other forms of anxiety management. Others regarded panic attacks as conditioned reactions to interoceptive cues and treated them by repeated exposure to these cues. Still others used cognitive methods.

In the past several years, substantial advances have been achieved in the development and refinement of treatments for panic disorder with and without agoraphobia (Barlow 1988; Brown et al. 1992; Michelson and Marchione 1991). For example, until recently, psychological treatments for panic disorder consisted largely of exposure-based interventions targeting agoraphobic avoidance. On the whole, these treatments did not address panic disorder directly, although some reduction in panic attack frequency was often observed after successful exposure-based treatment. Since the advent of the DSM-III-R (American Psychiatric Association 1987), in which panic disorder was separated from generalized anxiety and panic disorder with agoraphobia was reconceptualized as a variant of panic disorder, treatments aimed directly at panic attack reduction have been developed and evaluated. In general, these treatments have been successful in effecting clinically significant change in patients with panic disorder. Moreover, studies examining the comparative and combined efficacy of these panic-control treatments (PCTs) with pharmacological treatments have recently emerged in the literature.

Psychoanalysis and Psychoanalytic-Oriented Therapy

Psychodynamic psychotherapy in the treatment of panic disorder and agoraphobia awaits controlled trials, but case studies and uncontrolled clinical evidence indicate a role for this type of psychotherapy.

The psychoanalytic theory of neurosis has had a great impact on psychiatry in Scandinavia, and psychoanalytic-oriented psychotherapy has been considered the appropriate technique there for treating nonpsychotic anxiety disorders. According to Vangaard (1989), the therapeutic effort must include an elucidation of unconscious conflict, which might be resolved by means of insight, interpretation, and working through. With this resolution, the anxiety symptoms may disappear.

It is unclear how psychodynamic techniques for the treatment of neurotic states can be applied in treating panic disorder. Controlled trials of various psychodynamic techniques (such as support, interpretation, insight, and working through unconscious conflicts) are needed. There are a number of case reports of successful treatment of panic disorder through psychoanalysis or psychodynamic psychotherapy. These reports suggest that dynamic mechanisms alone may account for symptoms and that these alternative treatments can bring relief, sometimes as rapidly as medication or cognitive-behavioral therapy.

There have been no controlled clinical trials of psychodynamic psychotherapy, only uncontrolled case studies of small series of patients. Several case reports describe successful treatment of phobic patients with psychodynamic psychotherapy (e.g., Sifneos 1979). However, there have been few reports on the treatment of panic disorder. Malan (1976) reported three patients and Mann (1973) reported one patient who appeared to have met criteria for panic disorder and who were treated successfully with brief dynamic psychotherapy. In these cases, treatment focused on the interpretation of unacknowledged aggression as the central conflict. Millrod and Shear (1991) described three cases of panic disorder in which psychodynamic psychotherapy brought about improvement in symptoms within about 6 weeks. In these cases, panic disorder appeared to be triggered in the setting of growing independence and intense ambivalent feelings. In follow-up ranging from 2 to 5 years, none of the patients had a recurrence of panic disorder. Two case reports, by Zilber (1989) and Abend and Porder (1986), also described successful treatment with psychoanalysis of patients with panic attacks. Without control subjects, however, it is difficult to assess the significance of these findings.

Exposure-Based Therapy

To date, the primary modality in the psychosocial treatment of panic disorder has been exposure-based therapy (Barlow 1988). This type of treatment entails exposing the patient to anxiety-provoking situations (i.e., phobic stimuli). Although its mechanism of action is unclear (Barlow 1988), exposure-based treatment has been applied effectively in a variety of formats (e.g., situational [in vivo] vs. imaginal; gradual vs. rapid; therapist or self-directed vs. spouse directed). Reviews of the literature on exposure-based treatment have generally concurred that the format of gradual, therapist-assisted, situational exposure appears most effective (Barlow 1988; Michelson and Marchione 1991), although specific variations of this format may offer advantages in selected patients (see later discussion). Moreover, these reviews indicate that roughly 60% to 75% of patients with panic disorder with agoraphobia who complete this type of treatment respond in a clinically significant manner (Barlow 1988; Clum 1989; Jansson and Öst 1982; Michelson and Marchione 1991). Some exemplary outcome studies in which exposure-based treatment was used are included in the discussions of long-term follow-up and comparative outcomes.

Although most cognitive-behavioral researchers concur that some form of therapeutic exposure is a necessary element in the treatment of agoraphobia, various modifications in the delivery of this therapy have been examined in an effort to maximize treatment efficacy. One of the most extensively studied variations of the exposure format has been intervention in the interpersonal system of the patient by including the spouse in treatment. Treatment typically entails educating the spouse on the nature of agoraphobia and training him or her to serve as a "coach" in the patient's situational exposure exercises. This approach may have advantages. First, participation may facilitate between-sessions practice and practice after the active treatment phase. Such practice may enhance generalization of treatment effects because this format allows for therapeutic exposure within the patient's home environment and mitigates the possibility of dependence on the therapist. Second, in cases in which marital discord may potentially affect treatment response, either as a pretreatment predictor (e.g., Monteiro et al. 1985) or as a consequence of successful treatment (e.g., Milton and Hafner 1979), inclusion of spouses in treatment allows for potential resolution of difficulties if they arise. Possibly as a result of these features, this treatment has often produced dropout rates lower than those observed with other exposure-based approaches (Arnow et al. 1985; Barlow et al. 1984; Jannoun et al. 1980; Mathews et al. 1977).

In a study comparing 14 agoraphobic patients treated in a spouse-assisted program with 14 patients treated without their spouses, Barlow and associates (1984) found that the spouse-assisted group contained a significantly greater number of treatment responders at posttreatment assessment (86%) than the group not assisted by a spouse (43%). Both groups had attended 12 sessions of cognitive restructuring and self-limited exposure. Interestingly, there was a trend, albeit a nonsignificant one, for the treatment responder group to engage in a greater number of between-sessions practices than the nonresponders. Long-term follow-up of this study is described in the discussion of long-term psychological treatments.

In another well-controlled study in which spouses were included in the treatment of agoraphobia, Arnow and others (1985) evaluated whether the provision of a communications skills training package as an additional treatment component would significantly enhance treatment gains resulting from a standard spouse-assisted exposure protocol. Twenty-four agoraphobic patients underwent 4 weeks of spouse-assisted exposure, after which they were divided into two matched groups according to changes in their scores on behavioral measures of agoraphobia. One group received an 8-week communication training package that focused on communication patterns that may have potentially maintained agoraphobic symptomatology. The other group received 8 weeks of couples relaxation training. At both a posttreatment and an 8-month follow-up, patients who received the communications training package had a significantly greater response than the relaxation group on measures of agoraphobic symptomatology.

Relaxation Training

As with exposure-based treatment, relaxation training has been delivered in a variety of formats in the treatment of panic disorder with and without agoraphobia. Two of the most commonly studied formats are 1) progressive muscle relaxation (PMR; e.g., Bernstein and Borkovec 1973), which entails the systematic tensing and relaxing of the major muscle groups (often with relaxation-deepening components making use of deep breathing or relaxing imagery) and 2) applied relaxation (AR; e.g., Öst 1987), a modification of PMR entailing the rapid development and use of relaxation coping skills. AR has been used recently to alleviate panic attacks and anxiety experienced as a direct response to phobic situations.

In a study directly comparing variations of relaxation treatment, Öst (1988) compared the efficacy of PMR with that of AR to reduce panic attacks in 16 patients with panic disorder. Subjects were observed for an average of 19 months. Whereas both treatments were beneficial, 75% of the AR group were classified as achieving clinically significant gains at posttreatment assessment versus only 38% of the PMR group. All members of the AR group were panic free at the posttreatment assessment. Furthermore, of the 12 subjects available at follow-up, 100% who had been in the AR group were defined as improved to a clinically significant degree in contrast to only 25% who had been in the PMR group.

Öst and colleagues also conducted studies comparing AR with situational exposure in the treatment of panic disorder with agoraphobia (e.g., Jansson et al. 1986) and have found them to be of comparable efficacy. For example, Öst and co-workers (in press) found that the percentages of patients showing clinically significant improvement were 87% for AR and 73% for exposure. However, studies conducted at other sites that examined the efficacy of relaxation training have often achieved results less favorable than those obtained by Öst and colleagues. Many of these studies are included in the following discussions (e.g., Barlow et al. 1989; Clark et al., submitted for publication).

Cognitive-Behavioral Treatments

As discussed earlier, psychosocial treatments that are designed specifically to reduce the frequency of panic attacks have recently been developed and evaluated. These treatments have been developed in accordance with biopsychosocial models of panic anxiety (e.g., Barlow 1988; Clark 1986) that emphasize the role of such factors as catastrophic misinterpretations of the symptoms of anxiety and panic (e.g., misinterpreting palpitations as an impending heart attack), perceptions of uncontrollability of emotional states, hyperventilation, and learned (i.e., conditioned) associations between physical sensations and panic anxiety. Among the management techniques that have been developed are cognitive restructuring (e.g., identifying and challenging fearful cognitions associated with panic anxiety), breathing retraining, applied relaxation (discussed previously), and interoceptive exposure, which primarily entails the evocation of the somatic sensations associated with panic anxiety in a manner similar to the evocation of those sensations in situational exposure.

Several uncontrolled studies examining cognitive-behavioral panic management treatments have been conducted (e.g., Clark et al. 1985; Gitlin et al. 1985; Michelson et al. 1990; Newman et al. 1990; Salkovskis et al. 1986; Shear et al. 1991; Sokol et al. 1989). In general, these studies have produced converging evidence attesting to the efficacy of cognitive-behavioral treatments in ameliorating panic and its associated symptomatology. For example, Gitlin and others (1985) reported that 10 of 11 patients receiving cognitive-behavioral treatment directed at panic attacks were panic free after treatment. Similarly, Clark and colleagues (Clark et al. 1985; Salkovskis et al. 1986) treated 18 patients with panic disorder with and without agoraphobia with cognitive therapy and breathing retraining. Whether or not agoraphobia was present, the results indicated that treatment gains were maintained for up to 2 years (i.e., panic was virtually eliminated). However, this subject sample was restricted to panickers who experienced hyperventilation symptoms, and hence the generalizability of the results may be limited.

Sokol and associates (1989) implemented cognitive-behavioral panic-control procedures for 28 subjects with panic disorder with agoraphobia. Of the 26 who completed treatment, all were panic free at the conclusion of treatment, as were all 20 patients who were assessed at 3-month follow-up. Similarly, Michelson and co-workers (1990) used 12-week combination treatment with cognitive therapy and applied relaxation for 10 patients with panic disorder. At the conclusion of treatment, all subjects were panic free and met operational criteria for high end-state functioning.

Kabat-Zinn and colleagues (1992) looked at a meditation-based stress reduction program offered to a wide range of medical and psychiatric patients. Their study was conducted on 22 subjects with panic disorder with and without agoraphobia or general anxiety disorder, diagnosed by structured clinical interview, and used a within-subject repeated measures design (i.e., multiple pretreatment and posttreatment measures).

For 20 of 22 subjects, there was significant statistical and clinical improvement in anxiety/panic symptoms, depressive symptoms, and panic attack frequency was demonstrated at 3-month follow-up. Also, 10 of 13 subjects who had panic attacks at pretreatment were panic free at 3-month follow-up. This improvement was found to be maintained for 18 of the subjects who were followed at 3 years (Kabat-Zinn et al. 1992).

The intervention is consistent with cognitive behavior treatments in shared emphasis on noting sensations and thoughts without viewing them as catastrophic, use of stress-inducing situations as cues to engage in new behaviors, and use of homework assignments. The intervention differs from cognitive-behavioral treatments in that

1. Thoughts are identified as "just thoughts" rather than being positive, negative, or dysfunctional;
2. Observational skills are developed that foster a nonjudgmental awareness of thoughts and sensations, but without inducing, desensitizing, or monitoring these by any external data gathering; and
3. The intervention is presented in a nonpsychiatric setting to a heterogeneous group of patients as a way of living, rather than a specific treatment for anxiety given to patients homogeneous for anxiety disorders.

In a recent study in which a multiple-baseline, across-subjects, single-case design was used, Salkovskis and colleagues (1991) examined the efficacy of cognitive therapy in the treatment of seven patients with panic disorder with agoraphobic avoidance. Treatment for five subjects entailed brief (two sessions within a week) cognitive treatment designed to change catastrophic misinterpretations of bodily sensations. Treatment for the two remaining subjects entailed nonfocal cognitive treatment that did not address misinterpretations of bodily sensations. Nonfocal treatment failed to reduce the frequency of panic attacks and the belief ratings concerning the catastrophic nature of bodily sensations. However, four of the five patients treated with cognitive therapy showed a marked amelioration or elimination of panic attacks after two treatment sessions. A considerable decline in the rating of belief of catastrophic thoughts associated with panic anxiety was noted in all five patients. These results provided preliminary evidence that cognitive procedures directed at changing misinterpretations of bodily sensations can reduce panic attack frequency, whereas nonspecific cognitive interventions may not.

Comparative Outcome Studies of Psychosocial Treatments

In one of the few published studies to compare the efficacies of various psychosocial treatments directly aimed at reducing panic anxiety in patients with panic disorder with no more than mild agoraphobic avoidance, Barlow and colleagues (1989) compared the following treatment conditions: applied PMR, interoceptive exposure plus cognitive restructuring (PCT), the combination of relaxation with PCT, and a wait-list control (WLC). After treatment, more than 85% of patients in the two groups who used PCT were panic free compared with 60% of the relaxation group and 30% of the WLC group. Relaxation was associated with greater reductions on measures of general anxiety but also with greater attrition (33%). When the total sample was included in the analyses and dropouts were considered to be failures, approximately 80% of patients receiving PCT were panic free versus approximately 40% and 30% of patients in the relaxation and WLC groups, respectively.

Beck and colleagues (1992) recently completed a preliminary investigation to determine whether the efficacy of cognitive therapy for panic disorder is due to nonspecific factors. Panic disorder patients with and without agoraphobia were randomly assigned to either 12 weeks of cognitive therapy or 8 weeks of supportive therapy. When they were evaluated at comparable time periods (i.e., 4 and 8 weeks), the patients receiving cognitive therapy experienced significantly greater improvement than patients receiving supportive treatment, indicating that the effectiveness of cognitive therapy is not entirely attributable to nonspecific variables. However, this conclusion is somewhat limited by the fact that instruments to verify treatment credibility were not administered to patients. Thus, the possibility exists that between-groups differences in treatment efficacy were due to differences in treatment credibility.

In another recent outcome study involving cognitive-behavioral PCTs, Côté and associates (1990) compared the efficacy of 17-week therapist-directed treatment with minimal therapist contact treatment in 21 panic disorder patients without agoraphobic avoidance. After treatment, more than 82% of patients in both groups were panic free. Additionally, between-groups differences were negligible after treatment, indicating minimal therapist contact procedures to be a viable form of treatment for panic disorder, at least for patients at the level of severity studied. At a 6-month follow-up assessment, 90% of patients were panic free. These improvements were associated with a reduction in medication intake.

In addition to the studies reviewed here, several additional controlled trials comparing various psychosocial treatments for panic disorder are nearing completion (cf. Margraf et al. 1993). For example, Telch (cited in Margraf et al. 1993) reported initial findings from a study comparing a 12-session PCT package to a WLC in 71 patients with panic disorder without or with minimal agoraphobic avoidance. After treatment, the percentages of patients who were free of panic disorder were 85% and 30% for the PCT and WLC groups, respectively. In addition, Margraf and Schneider (cited in Margraf et al. 1993) are nearing completion of a study examining the outcomes of 82 panic disorder patients assigned to one of the following treatments: cognitive therapy, exposure (to external and internal anxiety-inducing cues), and combined cognitive-exposure and WLC. Cognitive therapy and exposure, respectively, were delivered without overlap in their components (e.g., exposure was carried out without cognitive reattribution of anxiety symptoms once those symptoms were induced). Interestingly, initial findings indicated that none of the active treatment conditions differed appreciably at posttreatment assessment, suggesting equivalence in treatment efficacy. Panic-free rates during this period ranged from 77% to 93% in these groups compared with 5% in the WLC group. Active treatment was associated with a total cessation of medication use in all patients who had used medications before treatment. The authors concluded that, whereas both cognitive therapy and exposure were effective in reducing the frequency of panic attacks and decreasing associated symptomatology, neither was a necessary treatment component (perhaps because they have similar mechanisms of action).

Finally, many of the studies examining the comparative efficacies of psychosocial treatments of panic disorder with substantial agoraphobic avoidance have been reviewed in previous discussions or are reviewed later. An additional relevant large-scale study has been completed by Michelson and others (1989), who reported the results of a comparative outcome study examining three treatments—graduated exposure (GE), GE plus cognitive restructuring (CR), and GE plus relaxation training (RT)—in 92 patients with panic disorder with agoraphobia. Patients in all groups received instructions for self-exposure (programmed practice). Of the 74 patients completing treatment, the percentages of patients achieving high end-state status after treatment were 86%, 73%, and 65% for the GE plus CT, GE plus RT, and GE only conditions, respectively. At 3-month follow-up, the percentages of patients meeting high end-state criteria were 87.5%, 47%, and 65% for the three groups, respectively. Analysis of clinical response in this study over a longer follow-up interval is currently in progress. In a similar type of study, de Ruiter and associates (1989) examined the relative efficacies of the following treatments in 49 patients with panic disorder and agoraphobia: breathing retraining plus cognitive therapy situational exposure and the combination of these two treatments. Whereas each treatment produced reductions in symptomatology on most measures (but not on panic frequency!), no evidence of differential treatment efficacy was noted. However, a comparison of the results of this study with others in the literature is hindered by the fact that standard outcome measures (e.g., panic-free status, high endstate functioning) were not reported.

Long-Term Psychological Treatments

Results of controlled studies examining long-term clinical outcome after psychosocial treatment of panic disorder with and without agoraphobia indicate that the majority of the patients who responded to treatment during the active treatment phase maintained their gains or showed continued improvement throughout the follow-up period (cf. T. A. Brown and Barlow, in press). In one of the more extensive follow-up studies that has been conducted to date on the long-term outcome of treatment for agoraphobia, Jansson and colleagues (1986) presented the results of a 7- and 15-month follow-up of 32 patients treated with in vivo exposure or AR. During the follow-up period, all patients were given self-exposure instructions. Although both groups had clinically significant improvement rates comparable to those in other outcome studies of agoraphobia treatment, these rates were significantly increased at both follow-up assessments. For example, whereas 59% of patients treated with in vivo exposure were improved to a clinically significant degree at the conclusion of treatment, this percentage increased to 65% and 71% at the 7- and 15-month assessments, respectively. Similarly, in the AR group, the percentage of clinically significant responders at the conclusion of treatment was 58%, increasing to 67% and 83% at the 7- and 15-month assessments, respectively. Only one relapse was recorded. In view of the continued improvement in many of the subjects in their study, the authors concluded that treatments for agoraphobia should contain a maintenance program of self-exposure for at least 6 months to ensure continued improvement or maintenance of treatment gains.

In a follow-up to the study of Barlow and colleagues (1984) described previously, Cerny and others (1987) found that a group of agoraphobic persons treated with spouse-assisted exposure had an increasingly more positive response than the group not assisted by a spouse at 1- and 2-year follow-ups, augmenting the between-groups differences observed at the conclusion of treatment. The continued improvement of the agoraphobic patients treated in the spouse-assisted format throughout the follow-up period is consistent with the results of several other studies. Those studies showed enhanced long-term functioning in patients treated with their spouses or significant others (Hand et al. 1974; Jannoun et al. 1980; Mathews et al. 1977; Munby and Johnston 1980).

Some of the findings pertaining to the long-term outcomes of uncontrolled trials of psychosocial treatments for panic disorder without substantial agoraphobic avoidance have been discussed earlier. Only a few controlled studies of the long-term outcomes of psychosocial treatments that specifically target panic disorder have been published to date, two of which were the Öst studies discussed previously (Öst 1988). Craske and colleagues (1991) recently reported 2-year follow-up results of the outcome study conducted by Barlow and associates (1989), described previously, who examined the comparative efficacies of applied PMR, PCT, and the combination of relaxation and PCT in the treatment of panic disorder without or with mild agoraphobic avoidance. Craske and others (1991) hypothesized that because more subjects in the relaxation group continued to have panic attacks at the conclusion of the original outcome study, between-groups differences might become more apparent over the follow-up period. Indeed, at the 24-month follow-up, when dropouts during the active treatment phase were included in the analyses and were presumed to be continuing to have panic attacks, 81% of the patients who received PCT only were panic free in contrast with 43% and 36% for the combination and relaxation groups, respectively. Patients maintained treatment gains or continued to improve on the majority of the remaining measures (e.g., general anxiety, depression). Craske and associates (1991) speculated that a dilution effect or a detrimental effect of the addition of relaxation accounted for the lower success of the combination group in comparison with the group who received PCT only.

These results compare quite favorably with the few studies reporting follow-up results of pharmacological treatments for panic disorder. In such studies, relapse of panic disorder has occurred in 70% to 90% of patients (Fyer et al. 1987b; Pecknold et al. 1988). Nevertheless,

Craske and colleagues (1991) observed that whereas the majority of subjects treated with PCT were panic free at 24-month follow-up, only 50% of those subjects met high end-state status criteria. These criteria reflect a combination of measures, including panic-free status, anxiety, avoidance, and functional impairment that would indicate whether a patient is essentially cured. This finding seemed to be a result in part of some subjects' continuing to have mild agoraphobic avoidance. Therefore, agoraphobic avoidance may have to be targeted separately in treatment because the elimination of panic attacks on its own may not be sufficient to ameliorate agoraphobic avoidance. These findings lend support to earlier assertions (e.g., Barlow 1988) that panic-free status, as a central outcome measure, may be an overly optimistic indicator of treatment success, because panic disorder patients who are free of panic at the conclusion of treatment often continue to experience substantial symptomatology (e.g., general anxiety, avoidance).

Comparative Studies of Psychopharmacological and Psychological Treatments

After having demonstrated the marked success of cognitive-behavioral treatment in reducing the frequency of, or in some cases eliminating, panic attacks in patients with panic disorder (e.g., Barlow et al. 1989; Michelson et al. 1990; Öst 1988; Salkovskis et al. 1986; Sokol et al. 1989), researchers have more recently devoted their efforts to comparing these treatments with current pharmacological treatments (e.g., imipramine, alprazolam). For example, Klosko and colleagues (1990) reported the findings of a study comparing the efficacy of their PCT (consisting of cognitive restructuring, breathing retraining, relaxation, and exposure to somatic cues) with alprazolam, placebo, and a WLC in 57 patients with panic disorder without or with minimal agoraphobic avoidance. As in the multicenter studies of alprazolam (e.g., Ballenger et al. 1988), daily doses of alprazolam were increased up to 10 mg with an average of approximately 5 mg. At the end-of-study assessment that was conducted while the patients in the alprazolam group were still taking their medication, 87% of the patients treated with PCT were panic free compared with 50% of those taking alprazolam, 36% of those taking placebo, and 33% of the WLC group. PCT was significantly better than placebo and WLC but not significantly better than alprazolam. Follow-up data are not available.

An important study by Clark and colleagues (submitted for publication) has been completed. In this study, 64 patients with panic disorder with or without mild or moderate agoraphobia were randomly assigned to one of the following groups: cognitive therapy (CT), AR, imipramine, or WLC. The CT treatment was similar to PCT (Barlow et al. 1989) and entailed identifying, recording, and restructuring catastrophic thoughts associated with the bodily sensations of panic and anxiety symptoms. Another element of this treatment was the induction of panic-like sensations via hyperventilation to demonstrate that negative predictions relating to the consequences of these symptoms are not borne out. The administration of AR treatment was similar to that described by Öst (1987). CT and AR treatments were delivered in up to 12 individual sessions over a 3-month period with the addition of no more than three booster sessions in the fourth to sixth months. Imipramine treatment was delivered in an equivalent number of sessions in the first 3 months, and subjects were maintained during the fourth to sixth months at the maximum dosage established in the initial 3-month period (mean = 233 mg per day); thereafter, the medication was discontinued gradually over 2 to 3 months. Subjects in all three active treatment groups received antiexposure instructions for the first 4 weeks of treatment, after which they received weekly self-exposure assignments. Subjects in the WLC group were randomly assigned to one of the three active treatments after 3 months. Assessments, including the evaluations of clinicians (unaware as to treatment groups), questionnaires, and patient self-monitoring, were conducted before treatment and at 3, 6, and 15 months.

The three active treatments were rated equally credible by the patients. The first of two multivariate analyses (conducted separately for panic-anxiety, depression, and cognitive measures) indicated that all three active treatments produced gains in the depression measures greater than those provided by the WLC group at the conclusion of treatment (i.e., 3 months). However, on the panic-anxiety measures, only the CT and AR groups achieved gains significantly greater than those of the WLC group; the imipramine group did not differ from the WLC in the multivariate analysis. Moreover, analyses of each of the individual panic-anxiety measures indicated that the CT group showed significantly greater improvement than the WLC group on all 17 measures at the conclusion of treatment; the AR and imipramine groups significantly differed from the WLC on 11 and 8 of the measures, respectively. Multivariate comparisons among the three active treatment groups revealed that subjects in the CT group achieved gains greater than those of the AR and imipramine groups on measures of panic-anxiety at the end of treatment and each follow-up evaluation. The AR and imipramine groups generally did not differ from each other on any of these measures; nor were there differences among all three active treatment groups in the measures of depression. Nevertheless, CT was superior to imipramine and AR on 12 of 17 measures of panic-anxiety (e.g., panic attack frequency and distress, Hamilton Anxiety Scale [Hamilton 1959], Beck Anxiety Inventory [Beck et al. 1988] scores, agoraphobic avoidance) and cognition (measures of fear of bodily sensations).

At the end of treatment, a significantly greater proportion of subjects treated in the CT group were panic free (90%) than those in the AR (50%), imipramine (55%), and WLC (7%) groups. However, at the follow-up assessment evaluations, rates of patients who were panic free did not differ between the CT and imipramine groups. For example, at 15 months, rates were 85%, 60%, and 47% for the CT, imipramine, and AR groups, respectively. On the other hand, treatment with imipramine was associated with significantly greater rates of relapse (40%) throughout the follow-up period than the CT (5%) and AR (11%) groups. Relapse was defined as emergence of three or more panic attacks within a 3-week period. Clark and colleagues (submitted for publication) interpreted these findings as a whole as supporting the superiority of cognitive therapy over other widely accepted treatment modalities in the treatment of panic disorder. Additional studies evaluating cognitive-behavioral treatments that target panic attacks directly are expected to appear in the coming years.

The studies by Klosko and associates (1990) and Clark and coworkers (submitted for publication) represent two of the small number of studies that have compared psychosocial treatments with pharmacological treatments for panic disorder without agoraphobia. Several studies examined the comparative and combined efficacies of therapeutic exposure and pharmacotherapy in the treatment of panic disorder with substantial agoraphobic avoidance. Most of these studies examined the efficacy of imipramine delivered in combination with some form of situational exposure (e.g., Mavissakalian and Michelson 1986b; Telch et al. 1985b). Some of these studies are reviewed in the next chapter. In one of the few studies to evaluate the effects of imipramine in the absence of in vivo exposure, Telch and colleagues

(1985a) compared imipramine plus instructions to avoid exposure, imipramine plus exposure, and placebo plus exposure in 37 patients with panic disorder with agoraphobia. After 8 weeks, patients in the imipramine without exposure groups had negligible improvement on panic, phobic avoidance, and anxiety measures, although a reduction in depressed mood was observed. In contrast, patients in the exposure groups, with or without imipramine, showed marked improvement on all measures. At the 4-month follow-up, the patients in the imipramine plus exposure group continued to show superior gains to those made by the other groups. Although imipramine seemed to potentiate in vivo exposure, certain caveats were noted, including rates of refusal (20%) and dropout (17% to 30%). Moreover, observed relapse rates in the literature, averaging 35% to 40%, reflect potential obstacles in the treatment of agoraphobia with imipramine (cf. Michelson and Marchione 1991). However, the dropout rate of 5% in the imipramine group of the study by Clark and colleagues (1992) study was well below the rates usually noted for this treatment, although relapse rates for imipramine (40%) in the latter study were consistent with previous rates. Clark and associates (1992) speculated that the use of a low starting dose and gradual dose titration beginning at 10 mg and increasing by 10 mg for the first 60 mg may have resulted in dropout rates much lower than those found in many other recent studies (Andersch et al. 1991; CNCPS 1992).

Combined Psychological and Psychopharmacological Treatment

As noted earlier, several studies examined whether the combination of pharmacological and psychosocial (e.g., situational exposure-based) treatment is more efficacious than the delivery of either modality alone in the treatment of panic disorder with substantial agoraphobic avoidance. The majority of these investigations have entailed the combination of imipramine with some form of therapeutic exposure (e.g., Agras 1990; Mavissakalian and Michelson 1986b; Telch et al. 1985a; Zitrin et al. 1983). In one of the earliest studies of this type, Zitrin and colleagues (1983) examined the efficacy of imipramine combined with either behavior therapy (imaginal exposure) or supportive therapy in a large sample of agoraphobic persons and persons with "mixed phobias" (e.g., patients with panic disorder without agoraphobia). Long-term results (i.e., at 2-year follow-up) indicated that the percentage of agoraphobic persons in each group meeting criteria for relapse (i.e., the return of agoraphobic avoidance) was 31% for imipramine plus supportive therapy, 19% for imipramine plus behavior therapy, and 14% for behavior therapy plus placebo, thus negating results that initially favored the imipramine over the "no imipramine" groups.

In another study examining the additive effects of imipramine and exposure therapy, Mavissakalian and Michelson (1986a) randomly assigned 77 agoraphobic patients to one of four groups in accordance with a 2 × 2 design (therapist-assisted exposure vs. programmed practice; imipramine vs. placebo). Although posttreatment results favored exposure, imipramine, or their combination over programmed practice alone, 2-year follow-up results ($N = 47$) revealed a slight reversal of therapeutic gain among imipramine-treated patients, whereas behaviorally treated patients tended to maintain treatment gains and further improve.

In one of the most recent reports on this type of study, Agras (1990) treated 100 patients with panic disorder with agoraphobia with imipramine or placebo, combined with either programmed practice (PP; self-assisted in vivo exposure) or instructions to avoid exposure. After an 8-week trial, subjects were then reassigned to 8-week trials of either PP or intensive group exposure (GE) while maintaining their original medication assignment. In the final 8-week phase, subjects continued medication and PP.

After the initial phase, PP was significantly superior to antiexposure instructions on several measures. Imipramine had little impact on outcome (except for depression), which the authors speculated may have been due to the gradual dose titration regimen performed in this phase. However, by the end of the third phase (24 weeks), a different pattern of results emerged: Using a global index of clinical outcome (which included measures of panic, agoraphobic avoidance, and depression), 59% of the imipramine plus PP subjects were substantially improved compared with 28%, 36%, and 14% of the imipramine plus GE, placebo plus GE, and placebo plus PP subjects, respectively. Thus, Agras (1990) concluded that the combination of imipramine and programmed practice was the most effective approach to the treatment of panic disorder with agoraphobia. As noted earlier, the importance of exposure as a basic therapeutic component in the treatment of panic disorder associated with agoraphobic avoidance is well established (cf. Barlow 1988). Indeed, in an earlier study, Telch and colleagues

(1985a) found that a group of agoraphobic patients receiving anti-exposure instructions showed no improvement despite the presence of imipramine.

To date, no studies examining the combined efficacy of pharmacological and psychosocial treatment (i.e., cognitive-behavioral, panic control-type treatments) for panic disorder without agoraphobic avoidance have appeared in the literature. Such studies will be of great interest in view of speculations about the possibility that concurrent medication use interferes with the action of psychosocial PCTs. For example, many newly developed treatments for panic disorder include a component in which panic attacks or panic-like sensations are evoked in the office to facilitate the learning of new methods of control over these experiences. Thus, the issue has arisen that psychotropic medications may prevent the elicitation of sufficient levels of anxiety in order for these techniques to be of maximal efficacy. To address this issue in a retrospective manner, Newman and colleagues (1990) assessed cognitive therapy without medication and with current antidepressants, anxiolytics, or both in 43 patients with panic disorder with or without agoraphobia. The majority of medicated patients (79%) were taking benzodiazepines either alone or with an antidepressant. However, the proportion of subjects whose medication dosage before cognitive therapy was considered to be of a therapeutic level was not provided. After a 12- to 16-week trial of cognitive therapy, 83% of medicated patients and 84% of nonmedicated patients were panic free, suggesting that concurrent medication use had no impact on outcome. At 12-month follow-up, 87% of both groups were panic free. Interestingly, only 35% of medicated patients were still using medications on a daily basis at the conclusion of treatment; this percentage did not vary when patients who used their medication only as needed were considered. At follow-up, the percentage of medication users had increased to 53%, but only 33% were taking medication on a daily basis at that time. The findings from several other studies have also suggested that, in panic disorder patients receiving psychosocial treatment, concurrent medication is not associated with a poorer outcome than no medication (cf. Margraf et al. 1993).

In view of the paucity of data evaluating the comparative and combined efficacy of newly developed cognitive-behavioral treatments for panic disorder and extant pharmacological approaches, a large-scale collaborative study sponsored by the National Institute of Mental Health was initiated recently to address this need (State University of

New York at Albany; Columbia University; Yale University; Payne Whitney Clinic at Cornell University). The interventions that are being evaluated include PCT, described previously, and imipramine in a 2 (presence or absence of PCT)×3 (imipramine, placebo, no medication) design.

The results from a small number of controlled studies that have specifically investigated the effectiveness of combined behavioral-pharmacological treatments in panic disorder with agoraphobia are summarized later. The pharmacological agent in all six published studies was the TCA imipramine. Behavioral treatments consisted of instructions and encouragement for self-directed exposure to phobic situations with or without therapist-assisted in vivo exposure sessions (Marks et al. 1983; Mavissakalian and Michelson 1986a; Mavissakalian et al. 1983; Telch et al. 1985b; Zitrin et al. 1980, 1983). As discussed in detail elsewhere (Mavissakalian and Jones 1990), four of five studies that compared exposure treatment with combined exposure plus imipramine treatment found that imipramine enhances the therapeutic effectiveness of exposure-based treatment to a statistically and clinically significant degree. Two studies compared imipramine with combined imipramine plus exposure treatment, and both studies strongly suggest that systematic exposure treatment enhances the therapeutic effectiveness of imipramine to a significant degree. In one study (Telch et al. 1985a), the experimentally interesting finding that "countertherapeutic" instructions curbing patients' entry into phobic situations would block the antiphobic and even antipanic effects of imipramine was reported.

The major practical implication of the mutually potentiating effects of imipramine and exposure is that combination treatment enhances the probability that patients will respond to treatment. There is, therefore, empirical support for combining behavioral and pharmacological approaches in the treatment of panic disorder with agoraphobia. Treatments induce significant improvement in the phobic dimension of this disorder, with the combined treatment being superior to the individual components. It is more difficult to provide a consensus summary on the differential antipanic effects of imipramine and exposure on the basis of these studies. In the best possible scenario suggested by the literature, the antipanic effects of exposure and imipramine behave in a manner similar to their antiphobic effects.

For the majority of patients treated with imipramine, therapist-assisted in vivo sessions may be unnecessary (Marks et al. 1983;

Mavissakalian and Michelson 1986). A combination of imipramine and instructions for systematic self-directed exposure may well be the most effective and cost-efficient method of combined treatments (W. S. Agras, personal communication, 1991). However, usual therapeutic antipanic doses of imipramine are required to confer therapeutic benefit during combined treatment (Mavissakalian and Perel 1985). Additionally, treatment should be continued for at least 6 months for maximal improvement (Telch et al. 1985b; Zitrin et al. 1980, 1983). The long-term effects of the combined treatments are hard to assess, but limited evidence (Cohen et al. 1984; Mavissakalian and Michelson 1986a) suggests that initial combined treatment has neither detrimental nor beneficial effects on the lasting improvement associated with behavior therapy. Therefore, combined imipramine and exposure may have the double advantage of maximizing patients' initial response to treatment and of protecting against high relapse rates after discontinuation of imipramine alone (Mavissakalian and Perel 1992).

Conclusions

Collectively, the preliminary results from the studies of psychosocial treatments reviewed here suggest that the gains achieved by these interventions match or in some cases exceed those obtained by the current pharmacological treatments for panic disorder. Rigorous studies on combination treatments have yet to be conducted for the most part. The utility of these psychosocial treatments is highlighted by recent data on long-term outcome that suggest that patients responding to these interventions tend to maintain or even build on the gains achieved during the active treatment phase, although more data addressing this issue are needed. One potential advantage of these treatments is that they allow the patient to learn specific coping skills that foster the maintenance or generalization of treatment gains. Whereas one potential criticism of this form of treatment (e.g., cognitive therapy) is that its administration requires special training and patient contact additional to that required for alternative treatments (i.e., pharmacological), the initial data pertaining to long-term outcome may ultimately override this concern. Moreover, with the establishment of effective cognitive-behavioral treatments for panic disorder, as well as the emergence of manuals and workbooks designed for self-directed treatment (e.g., Barlow and Craske 1989), attempts have been recently initiated to disseminate these interventions to non-clinic-based populations. These efforts have included the examination of the comparative efficacies of clinic- versus home-based treatments for panic disorder (Côté et al. 1990) as well as the evaluation of minimal therapist contact procedures for housebound patients with panic disorder and agoraphobia (McNamee et al. 1989). These studies have provided initial evidence that these treatments can be administered effectively in formats that do not require extensive clinical contact or training.

Finally, despite the substantial advances that have been achieved in the past 5 years, considerable work is still needed on the development and evaluation of maximally effective treatments for panic disorder with and without agoraphobia. This need is highlighted by the finding that a substantial minority of patients do not respond appreciably to any treatment, either psychosocial and pharmacological. Moreover, very preliminary data (e.g., Craske et al. 1991) indicate that panic disorder and situational avoidance may each require specific therapeutic attention, because the successful treatment of one (i.e., panic) may not generalize to the other. In addition, an important component of the future research agenda is to more thoroughly evaluate predictors of treatment response because these findings may provide useful insights on how to refine existing therapies to promote maximal treatment efficacy.

6   Clinical Practice Patterns for Panic Disorder

Patterns of Prescription and Use of Antipanic Medications

The term "pharmacoepidemiology" refers to investigations of the use of medications in the community. In recent years, an upsurge of activity in this field has occurred because of increased attention to the safety and toxicity of available medications. In the area of psychopharmacology, a large part of this interest has been prompted by increases in the use of psychotherapeutic medications since the 1950s and the possible medical, psychological, and social consequences of what now is perceived as a high rate of use.

With regard to the use of medications for therapeutic purposes, pharmacoepidemiology traditionally has concerned itself with the nature, extent, appropriateness, and consequences of drug prescribing in the general population. One view, which reflects concern about substance abuse, assumes that patterns of use for many psychotherapeutic medications are determined primarily by their pharmacological properties. According to this view, medications that have the potential to reinforce self-administration and to produce physical and psychic dependence will have higher rates of regular, long-term use. Uhlenhuth and colleagues (1992) challenged this position and presented evidence that the patterns of use of psychotherapeutic medications are determined primarily by the clinical characteristics of consumers (Balter et al. 1984).

Several national surveys have been conducted on the use of psychotherapeutic medications in the United States and other countries, including western Europe and Japan. The data from these studies indicate a rate of use of around 10% for anxiolytics, primarily benzodiazepines, in the United States; the rates in other countries range from 7% to 17% (Balter et al. 1984). Data from the United States indicate that a high percentage of persons who receive anxiolytics merit treatment by clinical standards. Conversely, only a small percentage of the general population with a clearly defined clinical need receives treatment with any psychotherapeutic medication.

General Patterns of Use of Benzodiazepines

The benzodiazepines, particularly diazepam, were the most frequently prescribed drugs in the 1970s, with a peak in about 1973. More recently, there has been a considerable decline in prescription and usage in part because of public concern about toxicity and dependence. Nevertheless, benzodiazepines remain among the most widely used medications for anxiety states, insomnia, tension states, and depression. About 50% of patients who receive medications in this class have a chronic medical illness; the medications are used as an adjunct in the treatment of their primary medical condition (Mellinger et al. 1984). Benzodiazepines are more frequently used than antidepressant drugs for panic disorder and even for depression (Klerman et al. 1992; Uhlenhuth et al. 1983).

Panic Disorder

Data from pharmacoepidemiological studies provide some information about actual clinical practice patterns in the diagnosis and treatment of anxiety disorders, including panic disorder. The data from these studies on panic disorder are limited in part because of the newness of the diagnostic category. Information dating before the 1970s is, for the most part, nonexistent. However, the data that are available from a number of sources (Uhlenhuth et al. 1983) indicate that patients with panic disorder have high levels of help-seeking behavior, in particular, high rates of treatment with and use of anxiolytic benzodiazepines (Uhlenhuth et al. 1984). The rates of use of sleeping pills, antidepressants, and in particular minor tranquilizers were quite high in persons with panic disorder or panic attacks. For example, 42% of patients with panic disorder and 32% with panic attacks had used minor tranquilizers in the past year contrasted with 14% of subjects with other disorders and 7% with no mental disorders. Several studies have data relevant to this issue: the 1979 National United States Survey (Uhlenhuth et al. 1983), the National Institute of Mental Health (NIMH) Epidemiologic Catchment Area Study (Regier et al. 1984), and the Cross-National Collaborative Panic Study (Buller and Amering 1991).

Data from the 1979 national survey are of considerable interest. Uhlenhuth and colleagues (1983) developed an algorithm for making diagnoses of selected disorders roughly in accordance with DSM-III (American Psychiatric Association 1980) criteria from the Hopkins Symptom Checklist-90 (Derogatis et al. 1974; Lipman et al. 1979), which is a patient self-report. With these algorithms, Uhlenhuth identified a group of patients from the 1979 survey with panic-agoraphobia and other DSM-III disorders, in particular, major depression. Of the various diagnostic groups studied, the prevalence of treatment with psychotherapeutic medications was highest in patients with panic-agoraphobia. Most of these patients (55%) were treated with anxiolytics, primarily benzodiazepines. They also were more likely to have used psychotherapeutic medications for prolonged periods of time.

The long-term use of benzodiazepines can be interpreted alternatively as a success or as a failure of treatment. On the one hand, success of treatment can be claimed for the use of benzodiazepines in the long-term treatment of patients with panic disorder to prevent relapse and to promote social functioning. On the other hand, long-term use can represent failure of treatment when a patient is not able to discontinue medication successfully. Although data on pharmacological treatments are not available from the 1979 national survey, the doses shown in research studies to be beneficial in blocking panic attacks are probably considerably higher than the doses used in clinical practice, even in the 1990s.

The pharmacoepidemiological data suggest that significant changes have occurred in physicians' prescription and patients' use of medication for the treatment of panic disorder and related conditions, particularly agoraphobia. Increasingly, medications such as benzodiazepines are viewed according to the medical model of treating a chronic condition over time rather than the "aspirin for a headache" model, which previously stereotyped anxiolytic pharmacotherapy.

Treatment Considerations in Clinical Practice

With the demonstration that there are effective pharmacological and nonpharmacological treatments of panic disorder, most clinicians tend to use a combination of treatments for a typical patient. Frequently, clinicians favor the type of treatment with which they are most familiar, psychologists using predominantly behavioral and cognitive psychotherapy techniques and psychiatrists, to a greater extent, emphasizing medication. However, most clinicians use a combination of behavioral exposure treatment, education about the illness and its treatments, and medication in varying degrees. Even the most pharmacologically oriented clinicians use at least some behavioral exposure as well as cognitive treatment techniques. Almost all effective programs incorporate exposure to phobic stimuli in some form or another. The emphasis varies from simple encouragement to homework assignments between sessions to having someone accompany the phobic subject into phobic situations, either a spouse, fellow phobic patient, or therapist. Most programs make use of educational techniques, including written and tape-recorded materials that emphasize education about the illness and various self-help techniques for managing anxiety in phobic situations. Cognitive therapy techniques, in which the characteristic catastrophic thinking of panic-agoraphobic patients is repeatedly challenged as unrealistic and unfounded, are used frequently as well, although to varying degrees. Cognitive therapy approaches vary from simple explanation of the concepts and unsystematic attempts at challenging these thoughts to direct extensive challenge as the principal mode of therapy.

Whereas most effective programs currently in use appear to include educational aspects, some programs almost exclusively make use of exposure therapy or cognitive therapy. These programs are administered primarily by psychologists and behavioral therapists and use in vivo exposure aids with varying degrees of sophistication and systematic organization. In this context, patients are often referred to a psychiatrist if medications are thought to be necessary. The extent to which nonpharmacological treatments are offered and administered appears to depend on patients' acceptance of this mode of therapy and its availability. Psychiatrists tend to use education and some systematic exposure to cognitive psychotherapy but rely heavily on medication to resolve the symptomatic difficulties in panic disorder. Because of its availability and administration, medication may be the most common form of treatment, at least in the United States. Extensive behavior or cognitive therapies are often reserved for patients who fail to respond to a combination of medication, simple behavior therapy, some cognitive treatment, and education.

Despite their obvious value, systematic studies comparing practical combinations of these treatments have not yet been performed. Practical treatment issues are generally resolved by availability and clinician and patient preference.

7   Summary, Conclusions, and Recommendations

Summary of Findings

Panic anxiety occurs in many different countries, with full-blown panic disorder having moderate prevalence and panic attacks having high prevalence. Panic attacks and panic disorder have far-reaching consequences in afflicted persons, affecting their quality of life and help-seeking behavior.

1. Panic disorder is a chronic disorder with wide-ranging effects on medical status and personal and family functioning.
2. It is a disorder with a relatively high prevalence in comparison with other serious medical conditions.
3. Panic disorder may be associated with an increase in mortality, possibly as a result of cardiovascular disease and suicide.
4. The efficacy of short-term treatment for up to 12 weeks with alprazolam, imipramine, and psychological treatment has been demonstrated. However, panic disorder is a chronic condition; accordingly, treatment decisions depend, for the most part, on results obtained after 12 weeks.
5. A high percentage of patients relapse after varying lengths of drug treatment if medications are discontinued. Differential diagnosis of types of discontinuation reactions is complex and often difficult to make.
6. Clinical and epidemiological evidence of the severity and chronicity of panic disorder indicates that long-term drug treatment is justified if short-term drug treatment does not have lasting effects after the medication is discontinued.
7. There are a range of treatments, pharmacological or behavioral, for panic disorder. There is no absolute indication for any one drug in treating panic disorder; the decision must be tailored to the individual patient. Benzodiazepines, such as alprazolam, might be chosen, for example, for a patient whose panic attacks are so disabling

that rapid relief is required. Imipramine may be the superior choice in a patient with current comorbid substance abuse whose risk of developing dependence on a benzodiazepine may be greater than that in a patient without substance abuse.

8. The rationale for long-term treatment rests on the evidence that panic disorder is a chronic illness—with substantial impairment, a high relapse rate after discontinuation of medication, and comorbidity with depression and other mental disorders. The use of effective medications in panic disorder conforms to the medical model of treatment and management of chronic illness, akin to the use of diuretics for the treatment of hypertension, steroids for the treatment of arthritis, or lithium for the treatment of bipolar affective disorder.

9. There is strong evidence that behavioral techniques produce enduring benefits in some patients with panic disorder with agoraphobia. For panic disorder without agoraphobia, there is accumulating evidence that behavioral techniques have enduring effects, without the relapse and recurrence associated with drug treatment. However, further research is required before the relative long-term benefits of drugs, cognitive therapy, or other behavioral therapy can be established.

Implications and Guidelines for Clinical Practice

As in all areas of medicine, the averages provided by science must be sifted, selected, and adapted to the needs of each individual patient. Science, in its present state, provides the information that several treatments for panic disorder are, on average, more effective than no treatment, but it provides little reason at present to believe that one is, on average, very much more effective than another. On the other hand, no one treatment is effective for every patient, and the treatments differ widely in terms of specific advantages and disadvantages. Psychological treatments are rather demanding and time-consuming relative to drug therapies, and not all patients will comply with them, at least not initially. However, their effects may outlast those of drug treatment once therapy is discontinued. For other patients, taking medication is frightening, and they will not do it, at least not initially. High-potency benzodiazepines act rapidly with a minimum of side effects, either initially or on long-term administration. Their primary drawback is withdrawal or rebound on discontinuation. Discontinuation effects can usually be managed satisfactorily if the clinician has patience, good diagnostic and patient management skills, and an understanding of the pharmacology of the benzodiazepines. Tricyclic antidepressants (TCAs) are slow to take effect and cause considerable discomfort for some patients initially and for others perpetually. However, once a patient is past the initial difficulties, TCAs have very few disadvantages other than weight gain in some patients. However, TCAs may be contraindicated in patients with certain medical conditions, such as heart block, narrow angle glaucoma, postural hypotension, or urinary retention. Monoamine oxidase inhibitors appear to be highly effective and to be tolerated almost indefinitely. Their main disadvantages are dietary restrictions, drug interactions, hypotension, and weight gain. Fluoxetine and other selective serotonin reuptake inhibitors have not been extensively studied but appear useful, at least for some patients.

Psychological treatments seem to be the best choice for non-depressed patients who will comply with them, because of minimum side effects and apparent long duration of benefit. In the presence of panic disorder and coexisting depression, a drug with both antipanic and antidepressant properties is usually necessary. For any patient in whom psychological treatment alone or medication alone proves insufficient, the addition of the other modality seems clearly indicated.

Future Research

Whereas substantial progress has been made in the past decade, a number of significant areas remain in which knowledge is limited. This limitation restricts the ability to make firm recommendations for clinical practice and public policy, particularly with regard to the comparative efficacy, safety, and long-term effects of available treatments for panic disorder.

The basis for treatment of panic disorder with medication, with its attendant risks, depends on the evidence for the chronicity of the illness and its impact on medical morbidity and longevity, social functioning, and quality of life. Therefore, further epidemiological and follow-up studies to confirm these risks are necessary. Because most follow-up studies conducted today are based on clinical samples, with the underlying biases inherent in such samples, follow-up studies using nonclinical samples are highly desirable. Most epidemiological studies have been cross-sectional, although 1-year follow-up data from the second wave of the Epidemiological Catchment Area study are available.

Whereas the quality of knowledge about the safety and efficacy of individual compounds is relatively good, our ability to make comparative statements is limited. The best comparative data are derived from the Cross-National Collaborative Panic Study, Phase II (Klerman 1992), an 8-week study that compared imipramine, alprazolam, and placebo.

Ideally, a long-term comparative study (6 months of treatment and 1 year of follow-up) of TCAs versus benzodiazepines should be conducted. Data would then be available about the comparative efficacy not only against the symptoms of panic disorder but also for improving quality of life, reducing social disability, and affecting help-seeking behavior and possibly medical morbidity. Few studies of long-term treatment have been carried out and almost all were uncontrolled, making valid conclusions limited. Several long-term follow-up studies of behavioral treatment showed low rates of relapse.

For both clinical judgments about individual patients and for public policy judgments on drug regulation, more knowledge is needed about the risks and benefits of treatment, especially in the long term. The potential benefits of long-term treatment derive from the chronic nature of the illness and the growing evidence of impairment in social functioning and quality of life. A reversal of these effects by long-term medication would be of considerable interest both to the individual and to society. However, evidence for the lasting value of cognitive and behavioral treatments for panic disorder with and without agoraphobia indicates that patients who relapse after drug treatment should be offered these forms of psychological treatment. Brief and economical methods of administering some psychological treatments exist for panic disorder with agoraphobia, but further research is needed to develop brief methods of cognitive therapy. Additionally, drug treatment should not be limited to the issuing of prescriptions; when medication is dispensed, advice should be always given on psychological aspects of treatment (e.g., reducing avoidance, coping with anxiety).

Most attention pertinent to treatment with benzodiazepines has been focused on dependence potential and discontinuation reactions. As knowledge of those clinical phenomena has increased, it has been established that, with gradual dose reduction (taper), the severity, intensity, and duration of these reactions can be considerably reduced in most patients.

At the same time, the potential risks associated with long-term TCA use, which include a small risk of convulsion, changes in libido, weight gain, and anticholinergic effects (constipation, dry mouth, and urinary retention), need to be acknowledged. Pending the availability of further evidence, it is recommended that clinicians be aware of the availability of a variety of treatments, both pharmacological and psychological, for short-term and long-term use and that, within the range of established treatments, patients and doctors be given considerable freedom of choice and an opportunity for individualization of treatment programs.

References

Abend SM, Porder MS: Identification in the neuroses. Int J Psychoanal 67(2):201–208, 1986

Adams PB, Weissman MM: Panic disorder and suicide attempts based on best estimate diagnoses of relatives. (submitted for publication)

Agras S: Imipramine and exposure in the treatment of panic disorder with agoraphobia. Paper presented at the Symposium on Pharmacological and Psychological Approaches to Panic Disorder, Göteborg, Sweden, January 1990

Alexander PE, Alexander DD: Alprazolam treatment for panic disorders. J Clin Psychiatry 47:301–304, 1986

Allgulander C, Lavori P: Excess mortality among 3302 patients with "pure" anxiety neurosis. Arch Gen Psychiatry 48:47–52, 1991

American Psychiatric Association: Diagnostic and Statistical Manual of Mental Disorders, 2nd Edition. Washington, DC, American Psychiatric Association, 1968

American Psychiatric Association: Diagnostic and Statistical Manual of Mental Disorders, 3rd Edition. Washington, DC, American Psychiatric Association, 1980

American Psychiatric Association: Diagnostic and Statistical Manual of Mental Disorders, 3rd Edition, Revised. Washington DC, American Psychiatric Association, 1987

Andersch S, Rosenberg NK, Kullingslo H, et al: Efficacy and safety of alprazolam, imipramine, and placebo in treating panic disorder: a Scandinavian multicenter study. Acta Psychiatr Scand 365:18–27, 1991

Angst J, Vollrath M, Merikangas KR, et al: Comorbidity of anxiety and depression in the Zurich cohort study of young adults, in Comorbidity of Mood and Anxiety Disorders. Edited by Maser JD, Cloninger RC. Washington, DC, American Psychiatric Press, 1987, pp 123–137

Arnow BA, Taylor CB, Agras WS, et al: Enhancing agoraphobia treatment outcome by changing couple communication patterns. Behavior Therapy 16:452–467, 1985

Aronson TA, Craig TJ: Cocaine precipitation of panic disorder. Am J Psychiatry 143:643–645, 1986

Aronson T, Logue C: On the longitudinal course of panic disorder: developmental history and predictors of phobic complications. Compr Psychiatry 28(4):344–355, 1987

Arrindell W, Emmelkamp P, Monsma A, et al: The role of perceived parental rearing practices in the aetiology of phobic disorders: a controlled study. Br J Psychiatry 143(2):183–187, 1983

Ashton H: Benzodiazepine withdrawal: an unfinished story. Br Med J 288:1135–1140, 1984

Ballenger JC: Pharmacotherapy of the panic disorders. J Clin Psychiatry 47:27–32, 1986

Ballenger JC: Drug treatment strategies: dosage and duration. Paper presented at the symposium on Panic Disorder: Strategies for Long-Term Treatment at the annual meeting of the American Psychiatric Association, New York, May 1990

Ballenger JC: Long-term pharmacologic treatment of panic disorder. J Clin Psychiatry 52 (suppl 2):18–23, 1991

Ballenger JC, Sheehan D, Jacobson G: Antidepressant treatment of severe phobic anxiety. Scientific Proceedings of the American Psychiatric Association 130:103–104, 1977

Ballenger JC, Peterson GA, Laraia C: A study of plasma catecholamines in agoraphobia and the relationship of serum tricyclic levers to treatment response, in Biology of Agoraphobia. Edited by Ballenger JC. Washington, DC, American Psychiatric Press, 1984, p 42

Ballenger JC, Howell EF, Laraia M, et al: Comparison of four medicines in panic disorder. Paper presented at the 140th annual meeting of the American Psychiatric Association, Chicago, IL, May 1987

Ballenger JC, Burrows G, DuPont R, et al: Alprazolam in panic disorder and agoraphobia: results from a multicenter trial, I: efficacy in short-term treatment. Arch Gen Psychiatry 45:413–422, 1988

Balter MB, Manheimer DI, Mellinger GD, et al: A cross-national comparison of anti-anxiety sedative use. current medical research opinion. JAMA 8(suppl):5, 1984

Bant W: Diazepam withdrawal symptoms. Br Med J 4:285, 1975

Barbaccia MC, Coste E, Ferrero P, et al: Diazepam binding inhibitor. Arch Gen Psychiatry 43:1143–1147, 1985

Barlow DH: Anxiety and Its Disorders. New York, Guilford Press, 1988

Barlow DH, Craske MG: Mastery of your anxiety and panic. Albany, NY, Graywind Publications, 1989

Barlow DH, O'Brien GT, Last CG: Couples treatment of agoraphobia. Behavior Therapy 15:41–58, 1984

Barlow DH, Craske MG, Cerny JA, et al: Behavioral treatment of panic disorder. Behavior Therapy 20:261–282, 1989

Beaconsfield P, Ginsburg J, Rainbury R: Marijuana smoking: cardiovascular effects in man and possible mechanisms. N Engl J Med 287: 209–212, 1972

Beaudry P, Fontaine R, Chouinard G, et al: An open clinical trial of clonazepam in the treatment of patients with recurrent panic attacks. Prog Neuropsychopharmacol Biol Psychiatry 9:589–592, 1985

Beaumont G: A large open multicenter trial of clomipramine (anafranil) in the management of phobic disorders. J Int Med Res 5:116ff, 1977

Bech P: Quality of life in psychosomatic research. Psychopathology 20:169–179, 1987

Bech P: Measurement of psychological distress and well-being. Psychother Psychosom 54:77–89, 1990

Bech P: Measuring quality of life: the medical perspective. Nordic Journal of Psychiatry 46:85–89, 1992

Bech P, Hjortso S: Problems in measuring quality of life in schizophrenia. Nordisk Psykiatriask Tidsskrift 44:77–79, 1990

Beck AT, Epstein N, Brown G, et al: An inventory for measuring clinical anxiety. J Consult Clin Psychol 56:893–897, 1988

Beck AT, Steer RA, Sanderson WC, et al: Panic disorder and suicidal ideation and behavior: discrepant findings in psychiatric outpatients. Am J Psychiatry 148:1195–1199, 1991

Beck AT, Sokol L, Clark DA, et al: A crossover study of focused cognitive therapy of panic disorder. Am J Psychiatry 149(6):778–783, 1992

Beitman B, Basha I, Flaker G, et al. Major depression in cardiology chest pain patients without coronary artery disease and with panic disorder. J Affect Disord 13(1):51–59, 1987

Beitman B, Mukerji V, Kushner M, et al: Validating studies for panic disorder in patients with angiographically normal coronary arteries. Med Clin North Am 75(5):1143–1155, 1991

Bernstein DA, Borkovec TD: Progressive Relaxation Training. Champaign, IL, Research Press, 1973

Biederman J: Psychiatric correlates of behavioral inhibition in young children of parents with and without psychiatric disorders. Arch Gen Psychiatry 47(1):21–26, 1990

Blair R, Gilroy JM, Pilkington F: Some observations on outpatient psychotherapy with a follow-up of 235 cases. Br Med J 1: 318–321, 1957

Bland RC, Newman SC, Orn H: Epidemiology of psychiatric disorders in Edmonton. Acta Psychiatr Scand 77 (suppl 338):7–80, 1988

Bowden CL, Fisher JG: Safety and efficacy of long-term diazepam therapy. South Med J 73:1581–1584, 1980

Brecher M: Review and evaluation of clinical data original NDA 19-906 (pending) clomipramine (Anafranil). Summit, NJ, Ciba Geigy Co, 1989

Brier A, Charney D, Heninger G: Major depression in patients with agoraphobia and panic disorder. Arch Gen Psychiatry 41(12):1129–1135, 1984

Brier A, Charney D, Heninger G: The diagnostic validity of anxiety disorders and their relationship to depressive illness. Am J Psychiatry 142(7):787–797, 1985

Brier A, Charney DS, Heninger GR: Agoraphobia with panic attacks: development, diagnostic stability, and course of illness. Arch Gen Psychiatry 45:423–428, 1986

Britton KT, Page M, Baldwin H, et al: Anxiolytic activity of steroid anesthetic alphaxalone. J Pharmacol Exp Ther 258(1):124–129, 1991

Brown TA, Barlow DH: Panic disorder and panic disorder with agoraphobia, in Principles and Practice of Relapse Prevention. Edited by Wilson PH. New York, Guilford, pp 191–212

Brown TA, Hertz RM, Barlow DH: New developments in cognitive-behavioral treatment of anxiety disorders, in American Psychiatric Press Review of Psychiatry, Vol 11. Edited by Tasman A. Washington, DC, American Psychiatric Press, 1992

Burrows GD: Managing long-term therapy for panic disorder. J Clin Psychiatry 51:9–11, 1990a

Burrows GD: Long-term treatment of panic disorder. Paper presented at the Symposium on Panic and Anxiety: A Decade of Progress, Geneva, Switzerland, June 21, 1990b

Clum GA: Psychological interventions vs. drugs in the treatment of panic. Behavior Therapy 20:429–457, 1989

Cohen ME, White PD, Johnson RE: Neurocirculatory asthenia, anxiety neurosis or the effort syndrome. Arch Intern Med 81:260, 1948

Cohn JB, Wilcox CS: Long-term comparison of alprazolam, lorazepam and placebo in patients with an anxiety disorder. Pharmacotherapy 4:93–98, 1984

Coryell W, Endicott J, Andreasen N, et al: Depression and panic attacks: the significance of overlap as reflected in follow-up and family study data. Am J Psychiatry 145:293–300, 1988

Coryell W, Noyes RJ, Reich J: The prognostic significance of HPA axis disturbance in panic disorder: a three-year follow-up. Biol Psychiatry 29(2):96–102, 1991

Côté G, Gauthier JG, Laberge B, et al: Clinic-based vs. home-based treatment with minimal therapist contact for panic disorder. Paper presented at the meeting of the Association for Advancement of Behavior Therapy, San Francisco, CA, November 1990

Craske MG, Brown TA, Barlow DH: Behavioral treatment of panic: a two-year follow-up. Behavior Therapy 22:289–304, 1991

Creed F, Guthrie E: Psychological treatments of the irritable bowel syndrome: a review. Gut 30(11):1601–1609, 1989

Crowe RR: Molecular genetics and panic disorder, in Neurobiology of Panic Disorder. Edited by Ballenger J. New York, Wiley-Liss, 1991, pp 59–70

Crowe RR, Noyes R Jr, Pauls DL, et al: A family study of panic disorder. Arch Gen Psychiatry 40:1065–1069, 1983

Crowe RR, Noyes R Jr, Wilson AF, et al: A linkage study of panic disorder. Arch Gen Psychiatry 44:933–937, 1987

Curtis GC, Massana J, Udina C, et al: Maintenance drug therapy of panic disorder. Paper presented at the 143rd annual meeting of the American Psychiatric Association, New York, May 1990

DaCosta JM: On irritable heart: a clinical study of a functional cardiac disorder and its consequences. Am J Med Sci 61:17–52, 1871

Deltito JA, Argyle N, Klerman GL: Patients with panic disorder unaccompanied by depression improve with alprazolam and imipramine treatment. J Clin Psychiatry 52:121–127, 1991

Den Boer JA, Westenberg HG: Effect of a serotonin and noradrenaline uptake inhibitor in panic disorders: a double-blind comparison study with fluvoxamine and maprotiline. Int Clin Psychopharmacol 3(1):59–74, 1988

Den Boer JA, Westenberg HG: Serotonin function in panic disorder: a double-blind placebo controlled study with fluvoxamine and ritanserin. Psychopharmacology (Berlin) 102(1):85–94, 1990a

Den Boer JA, Westenberg HG: Behavioral, neuroendocrine, and biochemical effects of 5-hydroxytryptophan administration in panic disorder. Psychiatr Res 31(3):267–278, 1990b

den Boer JA, Westenberg HGM, Kamerbeek WD, et al: Effect of serotonin uptake inhibitors in anxiety disorders: a double-blind comparison of clomipramine and fluvoxamine. Int Clin Psychopharmacol 2:21–32, 1987

Derogatis LR, Lipman RS, Rickels K, et al: The Hopkins Symptom Checklist (HSCL): a self-report symptom inventory. Behav Sci 19:1–15, 1974

de Ruiter C, Rijken H, Garssen B, et al: Breathing retraining, exposure, and a combination of both in the treatment of panic disorder with agoraphobia. Behav Res Ther 27:647–655, 1989

Dirks J, Schraa J, Brown E, and Kinsman R. Psycho maintenance in asthma: Hospitalization rates and financial impact. Br J Med Psychol 53(4):349–354, 1980

Dupont RL, Swinson RP, Ballenger JC, et al: Discontinuation of alprazolam after long-term treatment of panic-related disorders. J Clin Psychopharmacol 12(5):352–354, 1992

Dupont RL, Swinson RP, Ballenger JC, et al: Discontinuation effects of alprazolam: follow-up of long-term treatment of panic-related disorders. Report from the Cross-National Collaborative Panic Study (first phase). (submitted for publication)

Ehlers A, Margraf J, Roth W, et al: Anxiety induced by false heart rate feedback in patients with panic disorder. Behav Res Ther 26(1):1–11, 1988

Eitinger L: Studies in neuroses. Acta Psychiatr Neurol Scand 30 (suppl 101):5, 1955

Endicott J, Spitzer RL: A diagnostic interview: The Schedule for Affective Disorders and Schizophrenia. Arch Gen Psychiatry 35:837–844, 1978

Evans L, Kennedy J, Schneide P, et al: Selective serotonin uptake inhibitor in agoraphobia with panic attacks: a double-blind comparison of zimeldine, imipramine, and placebo. Acta Psychiatr Scand 73(1):49–53, 1986

Fabre LF, McLendon DM, Stephens AG: Comparison of the therapeutic effect, tolerance and safety of ketazolam and diazepam administered for six months to outpatients with chronic anxiety neurosis. J Int Med Res 9:191–198, 1981

Faravelli C: Life events preceding the onset of panic disorder. J Affect Disord 9(1):103–105, 1985

Faravelli C, Degl'Innocenti BG, Giardinelli L: Epidemiology of anxiety disorders in Florence. Acta Psychiatr Scand 79(4):308–312, 1989

Fava GA, Grandi S, Canestrari R: Prodromal symptoms in panic disorder with agoraphobia. Am J Psychiatry 145(12):1564–1567, 1988

Feighner JP, Robins E, Guze SB, et al: Diagnostic criteria for use in psychiatric research. Arch Gen Psychiatry 26:57–63, 1972

Feinstein AR: The pre-therapeutic classification of comorbidity in chronic disease. Journal of Chronic Disease 23:455–468, 1970

Fink M, Klein DF, Kramer JC: Clinical efficacy of chlorpromazine-procyclidine combination, imipramine and placebo in depressive disorders. Psychopharmacologia 7:27–36, 1965

Foulds GA, Hope K: Manual of the Symptom-Sign Inventory. London, England, University of London Press, 1968

Frank E, Kupfer DJ, Perel JM, et al: Three-year outcomes for maintenance therapies in recurrent depression. Arch Gen Psychiatry 47:1093–1099, 1989

Freud S: Obsessions and phobias: their psychical mechanisms and their aetiology (1895), in Collected Papers, Vol 1. Translated and edited by Strachey J. London, England, Hogarth Press, 1940

Freud S: Hemmung, Symptom und Angst (1926) in Gesammelte Werke XIV. London, England, Imago Publishing, 1948, pp 111–206

Freud S: On the grounds for detaching a particular syndrome from neurasthenia under the description "anxiety neurosis," in Standard Edition of the Complete Psychological Works of Sigmund Freud, Vol 3. London, England, Hogarth Press, 1962

Freud S: Mourning and melancholia (1917), in The Standard Edition of the Complete Psychological Works of Sigmund Freud, Vol 14. Translated and edited by Strachey J. London, England, Hogarth Press, 1963

Friedel RO: The therapeutic value, limitations and hazards of treatment of psychiatric disorders with benzodiazepines, in Handbook of Anxiety, Vol 1: Biological, Clinical and Cultural Perspectives. Edited by Roth M, Noyes R Jr, Burrows GD. Amsterdam, Netherlands, Elsevier, 1988, pp 385–397

Fyer AJ: Effects of discontinuation of antipanic medication, in Panic and Phobias 2. Edited by Hand I, Wittchen HU. New York, Springer-Verlag, 1986, pp 47–53

Fyer M, Uy J, Martinez J, et al: CO_2 challenge of patients with panic disorder. Am J Psychiatry 144:1080–1082, 1987a

Fyer AJ, Liebowitz MR, Gorman JM, et al: Discontinuation of alprazolam treatment in panic patients. Am J Psychiatry 144:303–308, 1987b

Gitlin B, Martin J, Shear MK, et al: Behavior therapy for panic disorder. J Nerv Ment Dis 173:742–743, 1985

Gloger S, Grunhaus L, Birmacher B, et al: Treatment of spontaneous panic attacks with clomipramine. Am J Psychiatry 138:1215–1217, 1981

Goodwin GM, DeSouza RJ, Green AR: Presynaptic serotonin receptor-mediated response in mice attenuated by antidepressant drugs and electro-convulsive shock. Nature 317:531–533, 1985

Gray JA: The Neuropsychology of Anxiety. Oxford, England, Oxford University Press, 1982

Greenhouse JB, Stangl D, Kupfer DJ, et al: Methodologic issues in mainte-nance therapy clinical trials. Arch Gen Psychiatry 48:313–318, 1991

Griez E, Van den Hout MA: CO_2 inhalation in the treatment of panic attacks. Behav Res Ther 24(2):145–150, 1986

Griffiths RR, Roache JD: Abuse liability of benzodiazepines: a review of human studies evaluating subjects and/or reinforcing effects, in Benzo-diazepines: Standard Use in Clinical Practice. Edited by Smith DC, Wes-son DR. Boston, MA, MTP Press, 1985, pp 209–226

Gross AJ: Observations on long-term administration of lorazepam in anxiety states. an open comparison with diazepam. Current Therapeutic Research 22:597–604, 1977

Grunhaus L, Harel Y, Krugler T, et al: Major depressive disorder and panic disorder. effects of comorbidity on treatment outcome with antidepressant medications. Clin Neuropharmacol 11(5):454–461, 1988

Hand I, Lamontagne Y, Marks IM: Group exposure (flooding) in vivo for ago-raphobics. Br J Psychiatry 124:588–602, 1974

Harding T: Clomipramine (Anafranil) in agoraphobia. J Int Med Res 1:425, 1973

Harris A: The prognosis of anxiety states. Br Med J 2:649, 1938

Harris EL, Noyes R Jr, Crowe RR, et al: A family study of agoraphobia. Arch Gen Psychiatry 40:1061–1064, 1983

Hasin D, Grant B, Endicott J: Treated and untreated suicide attempts in sub-stance abuse patients. J Nerv Ment Dis 176:289–294, 1988

Henauer S, Gillespie M, Hollister L: Yohimbine and the model anxiety state. J Clin Psychiatry 45:512–515, 1984

Herman JB, Brotman AW, Rosenbaum JF: Rebound anxiety in panic disorder patients treated with shorter-acting benzodiazepines. J Clin Psychiatry 48:22–28, 1987

Hibbert G: Ideational components of anxiety: their origin and content. Br J Psychiatry 144(6):618–624, 1984

Himle J, Hill E: Alcohol abuse and the anxiety disorders: evidence from the Epidemiologic Catchment Area Survey. Journal of Anxiety Disorder 5(3):237–245, 1991

Himle J, McPhee K, Cameron O, et al: Simple phobia: evidence for heteroge-neity. Psychiatry Res 28(1):25–30, 1989

Hirschfeld RMA: Panic disorder: diagnosis and course. Paper presented at the 17th Congress of Collegium Internationale Neuro-Psychopharmacologi-cum, Tokyo, Japan, September 1990

Hirschfeld RMA: The clinical course of panic disorder and agoraphobia, in Handbook of Anxiety Disorders. Edited by Burrows G, Roth M, Noyes R. Amsterdam, Netherlands, Elsevier, 1992, pp 105–119

Hoes MJ, Colla P, Folgerin H: Clomipramine treatment of hyperventilation syndrome. Pharmakopsky 13(1):25–28, 1980

Hollander E, Leibowitz MR, Gorman JM: Anxiety disorders, in American Psychiatric Press Textbook of Psychiatry. Edited by Talbott JA, Hales RE, Yudofsky SC. Washington, DC, American Psychiatric Press, 1988, pp 443–491

Hopper JL, Judd FK, Derrick PL, et al: A family study of panic disorder. Genet Epidemiol 4:33–41, 1987

Jannoun L, Munby M, Catalan J, et al: A home-based treatment programme for agoraphobia: replication and controlled evaluation. Behavior Therapy 11:294–305, 1980

Jansson L, Öst LG: Behavioral treatments for agoraphobia: an evaluative review. Clin Psychol Rev 2:311–337, 1982

Jansson L, Jerremalm A, Öst LG: Follow-up of agoraphobic patients treated with exposure in vivo or applied relaxation. Br J Psychiatry 149:486–490, 1986

Johnson J, Weissman MM, Klerman GL: Panic disorder, comorbidity, and suicide attempts. Arch Gen Psychiatry 47:805–808, 1990

Joyce P, Bushnell J, Oakley BM, et al: The epidemiology of panic symptomatology and agoraphobic avoidance. Compr Psychiatry 30(4):303–312, 1989

Kagan J, Snidman W: Infant predictors of inhibited and uninhibited profiles. American Psychological Society 2:40–44, 1991

Kagan J, Reznick JS, Snidman W: Biological basis of childhood shyness. Science 240:167–171, 1988

Kahn RS, Asnes GM, Wetzler S, et al: Neuroendocrine evidence for serotonin receptors hypersensitivity in panic disorder. Psychopharmacology 96:360–364, 1988

Katon W (National Institute of Mental Health): Panic disorder in the medical setting (DHHS Publ No ADM-89-1629). Washington, DC, U.S. Government Printing Office, 1989, pp 56–59

Katon WJ: Chest pain, cardiac disease and panic disorder. J Clin Psychiatry 51(5, suppl):27–30, 1990

Katon WJ: Panic Disorder in the Medical Setting. Washington, DC, American Psychiatric Press, 1991

Katon W, Roy-Byrne PP: Panic disorder in the medically ill. J Clin Psychiatry 50:299–302, 1989

Katon W, Hall ML, Russo J, et al: Chest pain: relationship of psychiatric illness to coronary arteriographic results. Am J Med 84:1–9, 1988

Katon W, Vonkorff M, Lin E, et al: Distressed high utilizers of medical care: DSM-III-R diagnoses and treatment needs. Gen Hosp Psychiatry 12:355–362, 1990

Katon WJ, Von Korff M, Lin E: Panic disorder: relationship to high medical utilization. Am J Med 92 (suppl 1A):7–11, 1992

Katschnig H, Amering M: Panic attacks and panic disorder in cross-cultural perspective, in Clinical Aspects of Panic Disorder. Edited by Ballenger JC. New York, Wiley-Liss, 1990, pp 67–80

Katschnig H, Stolk J, Klerman G, et al: Discontinuation experiences and long-term treatment follow-up of participants in a clinical drug trial for panic disorder, in Biological Psychiatry International Congress Series 968, Vol 1. Edited by Racagni G, Brunello N, Fukuda T. New York, Elsevier, 1991, pp 657–660

Keller MB, Yonkers KA, Warshaw MG, et al: Remission and relapse in subjects with panic disorder and panic with agoraphobia: a prospective short-interval naturalistic follow-up. Arch Gen Psychiatry (in press)

Kelly D, Guirguis W, Frommer E, et al: Treatment of phobic states with antidepressants. Br J Psychiatry 136:49–51, 1970

Kendler K, Neale M, Kessler R, et al: Generalized anxiety disorder in women: a population-based twin study. Arch Gen Psychiatry 49(4):267–272, 1992a

Kendler K, Neale M, Kessler R, et al: The genetic epidemiology of phobias in women: the interrelationship of agoraphobia, social phobia, situational phobia, and simple phobia. Arch Gen Psychiatry 49(4):273–281, 1992b

Kerr TA, Schapira K, Roth M: The relationship between premature death and affective disorders. Br J Psychiatry 115:1277–1282, 1969

Klein DF: Delineation of two drug-responsive anxiety syndromes. Psychopharmacologia 5:397–408, 1964

Klein DF: Anxiety reconceptualized, in Anxiety: New Research and Changing Concepts. Edited by Klein DF, Rabkin JG. New York, Raven, 1981, pp 235–263

Klein DF, Fink M: Psychiatric reaction patterns to imipramine. Am J Psychiatry 119:432–438, 1962

Klerman GL: Overview: the Cross-National Collaborative Panic Study. Arch Gen Psychiatry 45:407–412, 1988

Klerman GL: Depression and panic anxiety: the effect of depressive comorbidity on response to drug treatment of patients with panic disorder and agoraphobia. J Psychiatr Res 24(suppl 2):27–41, 1990

Klerman GL: Panic disorder: strategies for long-term treatment. J Clin Psychiatry 52(2, suppl):3–5, 1991

Klerman GL, Coleman JH, Purpura RP, et al: The design and conduct of the Upjohn Cross-National Collaborative Panic Study. Psychopharmacol Bull 45:407–412, 1986

Klerman GL, Weissman MM, Ouellette R, et al: Panic attacks in the community: social morbidity and health care utilization. JAMA 265(6):742–746, 1991

Klerman GL, Olfson M, Leon A, et al: Measuring the need for mental health care. Health Aff (Millwood) 11(3):23–33, 1992

Klosko JS, Barlow DH, Tassinari R, et al: A comparison of alprazolam and behavior therapy in treatment of panic disorder. J Consult Clin Psychol 58:77–84, 1990

Korn ML, Kotler M, Molcho A, et al: Suicide and violence associated with panic attacks. Biol Psychiatry 31:607–612, 1992

Krieg JC, Bronisch T, Wittchen HU, et al: Anxiety disorders: a long term prospective and retrospective follow up study of former inpatients suffering from an anxiety neurosis or phobia. Acta Psychiatr Scand 76(1):36–47, 1987

Kupfer DJ: Lessons to be learned for long-term treatment of affective disorders: potential utility in panic disorder. J Clin Psychiatry 52:12–17, 1991

Kushner M, Sher K, Beitman B: The relation between alcohol problems and the anxiety disorders. Am J Psychiatry 147(6):685–695, 1990

Lader MH: Hazards of benzodiazepine treatment of anxiety, in Handbook of Anxiety Disorders. Edited by Burrows G, Roth M, Noyes R. Amsterdam, Netherlands, Elsevier, 1992, pp 221–232

Last C, Barlow D, O'Brien G: Precipitants of agoraphobia: role of stressful life events. Psychol Rep 54(2):567–570, 1984

Leckman J, Weissman M, Merikangas K, et al: Panic disorder and major depression: increased risk of depression, alcoholism, panic, and phobic disorders in families of depressed probands with panic disorder. Arch Gen Psychiatry 40:1055–1060, 1983

Lee C, Kwak Y, Rhee H, et al: The nationwide epidemiological study of mental disorders in Korea. Korean Medical Sciences 2(1):19–34, 1987

Lelliott P, Marks I, McNamee G, et al: Onset of panic disorder with agoraphobia: toward an integrated model. Arch Gen Psychiatry 46(11):1000–1004, 1989

Leon AC, Shear MK, Portera L, et al: Assessing impairment in patients with panic disorder: the Sheehan Disability Scale. Social Psychiatry and Psychiatric Epidemiology 27:78–82, 1992

Lipman RS, Covi L, Shapiro AK: The Hopkins Symptom Checklist (HSCL): factors derived from the HSCL-90. J Affect Disord 1:9–24, 1979

Lydiard RB: Desipramine in agoraphobia with panic attacks: an open, fixed-dose study. J Clin Psychopharmacol 7:258–260, 1987

Lydiard RB, Ballenger JC: Antidepressant in panic disorder and agoraphobia. J Affect Disord 13:153–168, 1987

Maier W, Buller R: One year follow up of panic disorder: outcome and prognostic factors. Eur Arch Psychiatry Neurol Sci 238(2): 105–109, 1988

Malan DH: Frontiers of Brief Psychotherapy. London, England, Tavistock, 1976

Mann J: Time-Limited Psychotherapy. Cambridge, MA, Harvard University Press, 1973

Manu P, Matthews DA, Lane TJ: Panic disorder among patients with chronic fatigue. South Med J 84(4):451–456, 1991

Margraf J, Barlow DH, Clark DM, et al: Psychological treatment of panic: work in progress on outcome, active ingredients, and follow-up. Behav Res Ther 31(1):1–8, 1993

Markowitz JS, Weissman MM, Ouellette R, et al: Quality of life in panic disorder. Arch Gen Psychiatry 46(11):984–992, 1989

Marks IM: The classification of phobic disorders. Br J Psychiatry 116:377–386, 1970

Marks IM: Agoraphobia, panic disorder, and related conditions in the DSM-III-R and ICD-10. J Psychopharmacol 1:6–12, 1987

Marks IM, O'Sullivan G: Anti-anxiety drug and psychological treatment effects in agoraphobia/panic and obsessive-compulsive disorders, in Psychopharmacology of Anxiety. Edited by Tyrer P. Oxford, England, Oxford University Press, 1989

Marks IM, Grey S, Cohen D, et al: Imipramine and brief therapist-aided exposure in agoraphobics having self-exposure homework. Arch Gen Psychiatry 40:153–162, 1983

Marks IM, Albuquerque AD, Cottraux J, et al: The efficacy of alprazolam in panic disorder and agoraphobia: a critique of recent reports [letter]. Arch Gen Psychiatry 46:668–670, 1989

Martin RL, Cloninger R, Guze SB, et al: Mortality in a follow-up of 500 psychiatric outpatients. Arch Gen Psychiatry 42:47–66, 1985

Maser JD, Cloninger CR (eds): Comorbidity of Mood and Anxiety Disorders. Washington, DC, American Psychiatric Press, 1990

Massion OA, Warshaw M, Keller MB: Quality of life: panic disorder vs. generalized anxiety disorder. Am J Psychiatry (in press)

Mathews A, Teasdale J, Munby M, et al: A home-based treatment program for agoraphobia. Behavior Therapy 8:915–924, 1977

Mavissakalian M: Initial depression and response to imipramine in agoraphobia. J Nerv Ment Dis 175:358–361, 1987

Mavissakalian M, Jones B: Comparative efficacy and interaction between drug and behavioral therapies for panic/agoraphobia, in Handbook of Anxiety, Vol 4: Treatment of Anxiety. Edited by Noyes R Jr, Roth M, Burrows GD. Amsterdam, Netherlands, Elsevier, 1990, pp 73–86

Mavissakalian M, Michelson L: Relative and combined effectiveness of therapist-assisted in vivo exposure and imipramine. J Clin Psychiatry 47:117–122, 1986a

Mavissakalian M, Michelson L: Two-year follow-up of exposure and imipramine treatment of agoraphobia. Am J Psychiatry 143:1106–1112, 1986b

Mavissakalian M, Perel J: Imipramine in the treatment of agoraphobia: dose-response relationships. Am J Psychiatry 142:1032–1036, 1985

Mavissakalian M, Perel JM: Protective effects of imipramine maintenance treatment in panic disorder with agoraphobia. Am J Psychiatry 149:1053–1057, 1992

Mavissakalian M, Michelson L, Dealy R: Pharmacological treatment of agoraphobia: imipramine vs imipramine with programmed practice. Br J Psychiatry 143:348–355, 1983

McNair DM, Kahn RJ: Imipramine compared with a benzodiazepine for agoraphobia, in Anxiety: New Research and Changing Concepts. Edited by Klein DF, Rabkin J. New York, Raven, 1981, pp 69–79

McNamee G, O'Sullivan G, Lelliott P, et al: Telephone-guided treatment for housebound agoraphobics with panic disorder: exposure vs. relaxation. Behavior Therapy 20:490–497, 1989

Mellinger GD, Balter MB, Uhlenhuth EH: Prevalence and correlates of the long-term regular use of anxiolytics. JAMA 251:375–379, 1984

Mellman T, Uhde T: Sleep panic attacks: new clinical findings and theoretical implications. Am J Psychiatry 146(9):1204–1207, 1989

Mellman TA, Uhde TW: Patients with frequent sleep panic: clinical findings and response to medication treatment. J Clin Psychiatry 51(12):513–516, 1990

Merikangas K, Angst J, Isler H: Migraine and psychopathology. results of the Zurich cohort study of young adults. Arch Gen Psychiatry 47(9):849–853, 1990

Michelson LK, Marchione K: Behavioral, cognitive, and pharmacological treatments of panic disorder with agoraphobia: critique and synthesis. J Consult Clin Psychol 59:100–114, 1991

Michelson LK, Marchione K, Greenwald M: Cognitive-behavioral treatments of panic disorder with agoraphobia: a comparative outcome investigation, in Emerging Issues in Assessment and Treatment of Anxiety Disorders. Chaired by Michelson L. Symposium presented at the meeting of the Association for Advancement of Behavior Therapy, Washington, DC, November 1989

Michelson L, Marchione K, Greenwald M, et al: Panic disorder: cognitive-behavioural treatment. Behav Res Ther 28:141–153, 1990

Miles HHW, Barrabee EL, Finesinger JE: Evaluation of psychotherapy with a follow-up study of 62 cases of anxiety neurosis. Psychosom Med 13:83–105, 1951

Milrod B, Shear MD: Dynamic treatment of panic disorder: a review. J Nerv Ment Dis 179(12):741–743, 1991

Milton F, Hafner J: The outcome of behavior therapy for agoraphobia in relation to marital adjustment. Arch Gen Psychiatry 36:807–811, 1979

Monteiro W, Marks IM, Ramm E: Marital adjustment and treatment outcome in agoraphobia. Br J Psychiatry 146:383–390, 1985

Moran C, Andrews G: The familial occurrence of agoraphobia. Br J Psychiatry 146:262–267, 1985

Moreau D, Weissman MM: Panic disorder in children and adolescents: a review. Am J Psychiatry 149(10):1306–1314, 1992

Moreau DL, Weissman MM, Warner V: Panic disorder in children at high risk for depression. Am J Psychiatry 146:1059–1060, 1989

Munby M, Johnson DW: Agoraphobia: the long-term follow-up of behavioral treatment. Br J Psychiatry 137:418–427, 1980

Murphy J: Trends in depression and anxiety: men and women. Acta Psychiatr Scand 73:113–127, 1986

Nagy LM, Krystal JH, Woods SW, et al: Clinical and medication outcome after short-term alprazolam and behavioral group treatment in panic disorder. Arch Gen Psychiatry 46:993–999, 1989

Newman CF, Beck JS, Beck AT, et al: Efficacy of cognitive therapy in reducing panic attacks and medication. Paper presented at the meeting of the Association for Advancement of Behavior Therapy, San Francisco, CA, November 1990

Nordahl TE, Semple WE, Gross M, et al: Cerebral glucose metabolic differences in patients with panic disorder. Neuropsychopharmacology 3:261–272, 1990

Norman TR, Judd FK, Marriott PF, et al: Physical treatment of anxiety: the benzodiazepines, in Handbook of Anxiety, Vol 1: Biological, Clinical and Cultural Perspectives. Edited by Roth M, Noyes R Jr, Burrows GD. Amsterdam, Netherlands, Elsevier, 1988, pp 355–383

Norton G, Cox B, Schwartz M: Critical analysis of the DSM III R classification of panic disorder: a survey of current opinions. Journal of Anxiety Disorders 6(2):159–167, 1992

Noyes R, Reich J, Clancy J, et al: Reduction in hypochondriasis with treatment of panic disorder. Br J Psychiatry 149:631–635, 1986a

Noyes R Jr, Crowe RR, Harris EL, et al: Relationship of panic disorder and agoraphobia: a family study. Arch Gen Psychiatry 43:227–232, 1986b

Noyes R Jr, Garvey MJ, Cook BL: Follow-up study of patients with panic disorder and agoraphobia with panic attacks treated with tricyclic antidepressants. J Affect Disord 16:249–257, 1989a

Noyes R Jr, Garvey MJ, Cook BL: Problems with tricyclic antidepressant use in patients with panic disorder or agoraphobia: results of a naturalistic follow-up study. J Clin Psychiatry 50:163–169, 1989b

Noyes R Jr, Reich J, Christiansen J, et al: Outcome of panic disorder: relationship to diagnostic subtypes and comorbidity. Arch Gen Psychiatry 47:809–818, 1990

Noyes R Jr, Garvey MJ, Cook B, et al: Controlled discontinuation of benzodiazepine treatment for patients with panic disorder. Am J Psychiatry 148(4):517–523, 1991

Noyes R Jr, Garvey MJ, Cook B: Controlled discontinuation of benzodiazepine treatment for patients with panic disorder [comment]. Am J Psychiatry 148(11):1621, 1992

Nunes E, Quitkin F, Berman C: Panic disorder and depression in female alcoholics. J Clin Psychiatry 49(11):441–443, 1988

Nutt DJ: The neurochemistry of anxiety: an update program. Prog Neuropsychopharmacol Biol Psychiatry 14:737–752, 1990

Nutt DJ, Cowen PJ: Diazepam alters brain 5HT function in man: implications for the acute and chronic effects of benzodiazepines. Psychol Med 17:601–607, 1987

Öst LG: Applied relaxation: description of a coping technique and review of controlled studies. Behav Res Ther 26:13–22, 1987

Öst LG: Applied relaxation in the treatment of panic disorder. Behav Res Ther 26:13–22, 1988

Öst LG, Hellstrom K, Westling B: Exposure, applied relaxation, and cognitive techniques in the treatment of agoraphobia. Behav Res Ther (in press)

Ottaviani R, Beck AT: Cognitive aspects of panic disorders. Journal of Anxiety Disorders 1(1):15–28, 1987

Parker G: Reported parental characteristics of agoraphobics and social phobics. Br J Psychiatry 135:555–560, 1979

Parker G, Tupling H, Brown LB: A parental bonding instrument. Br J Med Psychol 52:1–10, 1979

Pauls DL, Bucher KD, Crowe RR, et al: A genetic study of panic disorder pedigrees. Am J Hum Genet 35:639–644, 1980

Pecknold JC: Discontinuation studies: short-term and long-term. Paper presented at Symposium on Panic Awareness for Clinicians, chaired by Ballenger JC, La Costa, CA, November 1990

Pecknold JD, Swinson RP, Kuch K, et al: Alprazolam in panic disorder and agoraphobia; results from a multicenter trial, III: discontinuation effects. Arch Gen Psychiatry 45:429–436, 1988

Pecknold JC, McClure DJ, Appletauer L, et al: Does tryptophan potentiate clomipramine in the treatment of agoraphobic and social phobic patients? Br J Psychiatry 140:484ff, 1990

Perris C, Jacobsson L, Lindstrom H, et al: Development of a new inventory for assessing memories of parental rearing behavior. Acta Psychiatr Scand 61:265–274, 1980

Perugi G, Deltito J, Soriani A, et al: Relationships between panic disorder and separation anxiety with school phobia. Compr Psychiatry 29(2): 98–107, 1988

Pitts FN, McClure JN: Lactate metabolism in anxiety neurosis. N Engl J Med 277:1329–1336, 1967

Pohl R, Yeregani VK, Balon R, et al: The jitteriness syndrome in panic disorder patients treated with antidepressants. J Clin Psychiatry 49(3):100–104, 1988

Priest RG: The homeless person and the psychiatric services: an Edinburgh survey. Br J Psychiatry 128:128–136, 1976

Priest RG, Laffront I: British and French classification of mental disorders. Ann Med Psychol 150:313–317, 1992

Raskin A: Role of depression in the antipanic effects of antidepressant drugs, in Clinical Aspects of Panic Disorder. Edited by Ballenger JC. New York, Alan R Liss, 1990, pp 169–180

Regier DA, Myers JK, Kramer M, et al: The NIMH Epidemiologic Catchment Area Program: historical context, major obstacles, and study population characteristics. Arch Gen Psychiatry 41:934–941, 1984

Reich J, Noyes R, Troughton E: Dependent personality disorder associated with phobic avoidance in patients with panic disorder. Am J Psychiatry 144:323–326, 1987

Rickels K, Case G, Downing RG, et al: Long-term diazepam therapy and clinical outcome. JAMA 250:767–771, 1983

Rickels K, Schweizer E, Osanalosi, et al: Long-term treatment of anxiety and risk of withdrawal. Arch Gen Psychiatry 45:444–450, 1988

Rickels K, London J, Fox I, et al: Adinazolam, diazepam, imipramine and placebo in major depressive disorder: a controlled study. Pharmacopsychiatry 24:127–131, 1991

Robins E, Guze S: Establishment of diagnostic validity in psychiatric illness: its application to schizophrenia. Am J Psychiatry 126:107–111, 1970

Robins LN, Regier DA (eds): Psychiatric Disorders in America: The ECA Study. New York, Free Press, 1991

Robins LN, Helzer JE, Croughan JL: Renard Diagnostic Interview. St. Louis, MO, Washington University School of Medicine, 1977

Robins LN, Helzer JE, Croughan J, et al: National Institute of Mental Health Diagnostic Interview Schedule: its history, characteristics, and validity. Arch Gen Psychiatry 38:381–389, 1981

Rogers MP, White K, Warshaw MG, et al: The relationship between anxiety disorders and medical illnesses. Psychosom Med 53:219–220, 1991

Rosenbaum JF: New uses for clonazepam in psychiatry. J Clin Psychiatry 48 (suppl 3), 1987

Rosenbaum J, Biederman J, Bolduc EA, et al: Comorbidity of parental anxiety disorders as risk for childhood-onset anxiety in inhibited children. Am J Psychiatry 149:475–481, 1992

Roth M: The phobic anxiety-depersonalization syndrome and some general aetiological problems in psychiatry. J Neuropsychiatry 1:293–306, 1960

Roth M, Argyle N: Anxiety, panic and phobic disorders: an overview. Key Biscayne Conference on Anxiety Disorders, Panic Attacks and Phobias (1982, Key Biscayne, Florida). J Psychiatr Res 22(suppl 1):33–54, 1988

Roy-Byrne P, Lydiard B: New developments in the psychopharmacologic treatment of anxiety, in Anxiety: New Findings for the Clinician. Edited by Roy-Byrne P. Washington, DC, American Psychiatric Association, 1989, pp 149–178

Roy-Byrne P, Geraci M, Uhde T: Life events and the onset of panic disorder. Am J Psychiatry 143(11):1424–1427, 1986

Roy-Byrne P, Ashley EA, Carr J: Personality and the anxiety disorders: a review of clinical findings, in Handbook of Anxiety, Vol 2: The Phenomenology of Anxiety. Edited by Noyes R, Roth M, Burrows GD. Amsterdam, Netherlands, Elsevier, 1988

Roy-Byrne PP, Cowley DS, Greenblatt DJ, et al: Reduced benzodiazepine sensitivity in panic disorder. Arch Gen Psychiatry 47:534–538, 1990

Salkovskis PM, Jones DRO, Clark DM: Respiratory control in the treatment of panic attacks: replication and extension with concurrent measurement of behaviour and pCO2. Br J Psychiatry 148:526–532, 1986

Salkovskis PM, Clark DM, Hackmann A: Treatment of panic attacks using cognitive restructuring without exposure or breathing retraining. Behav Res Ther 29: 161–166, 1991

Sargant W, Dally P: Treatment of anxiety states by antidepressant drugs. Br Med J 1:6–9, 1962

Schatzberg AF, Ballenger JC: Decisions for the clinician in the treatment of panic disorder: when to treat, which treatment to use, and how long to treat. J Clin Psychiatry 54 (suppl):26–31, 1991

Schneier FR, Leibowitz MR, Davies SO, et al: Fluoxetine in panic disorder. J Clin Psychopharmacol 10(2):119–121, 1990

Schneier F, Johnson J, Hornig C, et al: Social phobia: comorbidity and morbidity in an epidemiologic sample. Arch Gen Psychiatry 49(4):282–288, 1992

Schweitzer E, Rickels K, Weiss S, et al: Maintenance drug treatment of panic disorder, I: results of a prospective, placebo-controlled comparison of alprazolam and imipramine. Arch Gen Psychiatry 50:51–60, 1993

Sciuto G, Diaferia G, Battaglia M, et al: DSM III R personality disorders in panic and obsessive compulsive disorder: a comparison study. Compr Psychiatry 32(5):450–457, 1991

Sethy VH, Hodges DH: Alprazolam in biochemical model of depression. Biochem Pharmacol 31:3155–3157, 1982

Shear MK, Ball G, Fitzpatrick M, et al: Cognitive-behavioral therapy for panic: an open study. J Nerv Ment Dis 179:467–471, 1991

Sheehan DV: Current views on the treatment of panic and phobic disorders. Drug Ther Hosp 7:74–93, 1982

Sheehan DV: The Anxiety Disease. New York, Scribners, 1983

Sheehan DV: One-year follow-up of patients with panic disorder, and withdrawal from long-term antipanic medication, in Program and Abstracts of the Panic Disorder Biological Research Workshop, Washington, DC, April 1986

Sheehan DV, Ballenger JC, Jacobson G, et al: Treatment of endogenous anxiety with phobic, hysterical, and hypochondriacal symptoms. Arch Gen Psychiatry 36:51–59, 1980

Sheehan DV, Raj BA, Sheehan KH, et al: Is buspirone effective for panic disorder? J Clin Psychopharmacol 10:2–11, 1990

Sifneos PE: Short-Term Dynamic Psychotherapy: Evaluation and Technique. New York, Plenum, 1979

Silove D: Perceived parental characteristics and reports of early parental deprivation in agoraphobic patients. Aust N Z J Psychiatry 20(3):365–369, 1986

Sokol L, Beck AT, Greenberg RI, et al: Cognitive therapy of panic disorder: a non-pharmacologic alternative. J Nerv Ment Dis 177:711–716, 1989

Solyom L, Beck P, Solyom C, et al: Some etiological factors in phobic neurosis. Canadian Psychiatric Association Journal 19:69–78, 1991

Spier SA, Tesar GE, Rosenbaum JF, et al: Treatment of panic disorder and agoraphobia with clonazepam. J Clin Psychiatry 47:238–242, 1986

Spitzer RL, Endicott J, Robins E: Research diagnostic criteria: rationale and reliability. Arch Gen Psychiatry 35:773–779, 1978

Starcevic V: Relationship between panic disorders, agoraphobia, and personality disturbance: an overview of research findings, and pertinent issues. Psihijatrija Danas 23(1–2):57–70, 1991

Stavrakaki C, Vargo B: The relationship of anxiety and depression: a review of the literature. Br J Psychiatry 149:7–16, 1986

Stewart WF, Linet MS, Celentano DD: Migraine headaches and panic attacks. Psychosom Med 51:559–569, 1989

Tainey J, Pohl R, Williams M, et al: A comparison of lactate and isoproterenol anxiety states. Psychopathology 17:74–82, 1984

Taylor CB, Hayward C, King R, et al: Cardiovascular and symptomatic reduction effects of alprazolam and imipramine in patients with panic disorder: results of a double-blind, placebo-controlled trial. J Clin Psychopharmacol 10:112–118, 1990

Telch M, Agras W, Taylor C, et al: Combined pharmacological and behavioral treatment for agoraphobia. Behav Res Ther 23:335–355, 1985a

Telch M, Agras W, Taylor C, et al: Imipramine and behavioral treatment for agoraphobia. Behav Res Ther 23:325–335, 1985b

Tesar GE, Rosenbaum JF: Successful use of clonazepam in patients with treatment-resistant panic disorder. J Nerv Ment Dis 174:477–482, 1986

Torgersen S: Genetic factor in anxiety disorders. Arch Gen Psychiatry 40:1085–1089, 1983

Torgersen S: Childhood and family characteristics in panic and generalized anxiety disorders. Am J Psychiatry 143(5):630–632, 1986

Tucker WI: Diagosis and treatment of the phobic reaction. Am J Psychiatry 112:825–830, 1956

Tyrer PJ, Candy J, Kelly DA: A study of the clinical effects of phenelzine and placebo in the treatment of phobic anxiety. Psychopharmacologia 32:237–254, 1973

Tyrer P, Rutherford D, Huggett T: Benzodiazepine withdrawal symptoms and propranolol. Lancet 88:520–522, 1981

Tyrer PJ, Owen R, Dawling S: Gradual withdrawal of diazepam after long-term therapy. Lancet 1:1402–1406, 1983

Uhde TW, Boulenger JP, Vittone B, et al: Human anxiety and nonadrenergic function: preliminary studies with caffeine, clonidine and yohimbine, in Proceedings of the Seventh World Congress of Psychiatry. New York, Plenum, 1985

Uhlenhuth EH, Balter MB: Clinical variables in pharmacoepidemiology. J Psychiatr Res (in press)

Uhlenhuth EH, Balter MB, Mellinger GD, et al: Symptom checklist syndromes in the general population: correlations with psychotherapeutic drug use. Arch Gen Psychiatry 40:1167–1173, 1983

Uhlenhuth EH, Balter MB, Mellinger GD: Anxiety disorders: prevalence and treatment. Curr Med Res Opin 8 (suppl 4):37–47, 1984

Uhlenhuth EH, Matsuzas W, Glass RM, et al: Response of panic disorder to fixed dose of alprazolam or imipramine. J Affect Disord 17:261–270, 1989

Uhlenhuth EH, Balter MB, Mellinger GD: Clinical variables in pharmacoepidemiology. J Psychiatr Res 24 (suppl):15–16, 1992

van den Hout MA, Griez E: Cardiovascular and subjective responses to inhalation of carbon dioxide. Psychother Psychosom 37:75–82, 1982

Vangaard T: Panic: The Course of a Psychoanalysis, 1st Edition. Translated by Vangaard J. New York, WW Norton, 1989

Versiani M, Gentile V, Paprocki J, et al: Data about 508 cases of panic disorder and responses to treatment with alprazolam clomipramine, imipramine, and tranylcypromine, in Biological Psychiatry: Proceedings from the IVth World Congress of Biological Psychiatry. Edited by Shagass C, Josiassen RD, Bridger WH, Weiss KJ, Stoff DH, Simpson GM. Amsterdam, Netherlands, Elsevier, 1985

Villacres EC, Hollifield M, Katon WI, et al: Sympathetic nervous system activity in panic disorder. Psychiatry Res 21:313–321, 1987

Vyas I, Carney MWP: Diazepam withdrawal fits. Br Med J 4:44, 1975

Walker EA, Roy-Byrne PP, Katon WJ, et al: Psychiatric illness and irritable bowel syndrome: a comparison with inflammatory bowel disease. Am J Psychiatry 147:1656–1661, 1990

Waxman D: A clinical trial of clomipramine and diazepam in the treatment of phobic and obsessional illness. J Int Med Res 5:99–110, 1977

Weissman MM: The epidemiology of panic disorder and agoraphobia, in American Psychiatric Association Annual Review of Psychiatry, Vol 7. Edited by Hales RE, Frances AJ. Washington, DC, American Psychiatric Press, 1988, pp 54–66

Weissman MM: Family genetic studies of panic disorder. Paper presented at the Conference on Panic and Anxiety: A Decade of Progress, Geneva, Switzerland, June 1990

Weissman MM: Panic disorder: impact on quality of life. J Clin Psychiatry 52(2):6–9, 1991

Weissman MM: Family genetic studies of panic disorder. J Psychiatr Res (in press)

Weissman MM, Klerman GL, Markowitz JS, et al: Suicidal ideation and suicide attempts in panic disorder and attacks. N Engl J Med 321:1209–1214, 1989

Weissman MM, Markowitz JS, Ouellette R, et al: Panic disorder and cardio-vascular/cerebrovascular problems: results from a community survey. Am J Psychiatry 147:1504–1508, 1990

Wells K, Burnam M, Leake B, et al: Agreement between face to face and telephone administered versions of the depression section of the NIMH Diagnostic Interview Schedule. J Psychiatric Res 22(3):207–220, 1988

Wells KB, Stewart AL, Hays RD, et al: The functioning and well-being of depressed patients: results from the Medical Outcome Study. JAMA 262:914–919, 1989

West ED, Dally PJ: Effect of iproniazid in depressive syndromes. BMJ 1:1491–1494, 1959

Westphal C: Die Agoraphobie, eine neuropathische Erscheinung. Archives of Psychiatric Nervenkrankh 3:138–161, 1872

Wheeler ED, White PD, Reed EW, et al: Neurocirculatory asthenia: a 20-year follow-up study of 173 patients. JAMA 142:878–889, 1950

Wing JK, Cooper JE, Sartorius N: Measurement and Classification of Psychiatric Symptoms: An Instructional Manual for the PSE and CATEGO Program. New York, Cambridge University Press, 1974

Wittchen HU, Ahmoi EC, Von ZD, et al: Lifetime and six month prevalence of mental disorders in the Munich Follow Up Study. Eur Arch Psychiatry Clin Neurosci 241(4):247–258, 1992

World Health Organization: International Classification of Diseases, 9th Edition. Geneva, Switzerland, World Health Organization, 1978

World Health Organization: Draft of the International Classification of Diseases and Related Health Problems, 10th Edition. Geneva, Switzerland, World Health Organization, 1990

World Health Organization: International Classification of Diseases and Related Health Problems, 10th Edition. Geneva, Switzerland, World Health Organization, 1992

Wulsin LR, Hillard JR, Grier P, et al: Screening emergency room patients with atypical chest pain for depression and panic disorder. Int J Psychiatry Med 18(4):315–323, 1988

Zandbergen J, Pols H, Fernandez I, et al: An analysis of panic symptoms during hypercarbia compared to hypocarbia in patients with panic anxiety. J Affective Disord 23(3):131–136, 1991

Zilber N, Schufman A, Lerner Y: Mortality among psychiatric outpatients: the group at risk. Acta Psychiatr Scand 79:248–256, 1989

Zitrin CM, Klein DF, Woerner MG: Treatment of agoraphobia with group exposure in vivo and imipramine. Arch Gen Psychiatry 37:63–72, 1980

Zitrin CM, Klein DF, Woerner MG, et al: Treatment of phobias, I: Comparison of imipramine hydrochloride and placebo. Arch Gen Psychiatry 40:125–138, 1983

Selected Readings

Allgulander C, Fisher LD: Clinical predictors of completed suicide and repeated self-poisoning in 8895 self-poisoning patients. Eur Arch Psychiatry Neurol Sci 239:270–276, 1990

Allsopp LF, Cooper GL, Poole PH: Clomipramine and diazepam in the treatment of agoraphobia and social phobia in general practice. Curr Med Res Opin 9:64–70, 1984

American Psychiatric Association: Task Force on Benzodiazepine Dependence, Toxicity and Abuse. Washington, DC, American Psychiatric Association, 1990

Amering M, Katschnig H: Long-term fate of specific agoraphobic fears in panic disorder. Paper presented at the annual meeting of the American Psychiatric Association, New Orleans, LA, May 1991

Angst J, Dobler M: The Zurich study. Eur Arch Psychiatry Neurol Sci 235:171–178, 1985

Ballenger JC: Drug treatment of panic disorder and agoraphobia. In CME Syllabus and Proceedings Summary of the 140th Annual Meeting of the American Psychiatric Association, Chicago, IL, 1987

Ballenger JC: The clinical use of carbamazepine in affective disorders. J Clin Psychiatry 49:13–21, 1988

Ballenger JC (ed): Clinical Aspects of Panic Disorder. New York, Alan R Liss, 1990a

Ballenger JC: Efficacy of benzodiazepines in panic disorder and agoraphobia. J Psychiatr Res 24:15–25, 1990b

Ballenger JC (ed): Neurobiology of Anxiety. New York, Alan R Liss, 1990c

Barbaccia M, Costa E, Ferrero P, et al: Diazepam binding inhibitor. a brain neuropeptide present in human spinal fluid. studies in depression, schizophrenia, and Alzheimer's disease. Arch Gen Psychiatry 43(12):1143–1147, 1986

Barlow DH: Long-term outcome for patients with panic disorder treated with cognitive-behavioral therapy. J Clin Psychiatry 51:17–23, 1990

Beard GM: A Practical Treatise on Nervous Exhaustion (Neurasthenia): Its Symptoms, Nature, Sequences, Treatment. New York, Wood, 1880

Beaudry P, Fontaine R, Chouinard G: Bromazepam, another high-potency benzodiazepine, for panic attacks. Am J Psychiatry 141:464–465, 1984

Bech P: Quality of life measurement in the medical setting. International Journal of Methods in Psychiatric Research 2:139–144, 1992

Beck AT: Cognitive approaches to panic disorder: theory and therapy, in Panic: Psychological Perspectives. Edited by Rachman S, Maser J. Hillsdale, NJ, Erlbaum, 1988

Brown JL, Hauge KJ: A review of alprazolam withdrawal. Drug Intell Clin Pharm 20:837–841, 1986

Brown S, Irwin M, Schuckit M: Changes in anxiety among abstinent male alcoholics. J Stud Alcohol 52(1):55–61, 1991

Buigues J, Vallejo J: Therapeutic response to phenelzine in patients with panic disorder and agoraphobia with panic attacks. J Clin Psychiatry 48:55–59, 1987

Buller R, Amering M: Follow-up in subtypes of panic disorder. Paper presented at the 5th World Congress of Biological Psychiatry, Florence, Italy, June 1991

Buller R, Maier W, Benkert O: Clinical subtypes in panic disorder: their descriptive and prospective validity. J Affect Disord 11(2):105–114, 1986

Busto U, Sellers EM: Pharmacokinetic determinants of drug abuse and dependence: a conceptual perspective. Clin Pharmacokinet 11:144–153, 1986

Busto U, Sellers EM, Naranjo CA, et al: Withdrawal reaction after long-term therapeutic use of benzodiazepines. N Engl J Med 315:854–859, 1986

Cameron O, Thyer B, Nesse R, Curtis G: Symptom profiles of patients with DSM III anxiety disorders. Am J Psychiatry 143(9):1132–1137, 1986

Canino GJ, Bird HR, Shrout PE, et al: The prevalence of specific psychiatric disorders in Puerto Rico. Arch Gen Psychiatry 44(8):727–735, 1987

Cassano GB, Petracca A, Perugi G, et al: Clomipramine for panic disorder: the first 10 weeks of a long-term comparison with imipramine. J Affect Disord 14:123–127, 1988

Cassem EH: Depression and anxiety secondary to medical illness. Psychiatr Clin North Am 13(4):597–612, 1990

Cerny JA, Barlow DH, Craske MG, et al: Couples treatment of agoraphobia: a two-year follow-up. Behavior Therapy 18:401–415, 1987

Charney DS, Heninger GR: Abnormal regulation of noradrenergic function in panic disorder. Am J Psychiatry 43:177–189, 1986

Charney DS, Woods SW: Benzodiazepine treatment of panic disorder: a comparison of alprazolam and lorazepam. J Clin Psychiatry 50:418–423, 1989

Charney DS, Heninger GR, Breier A: Noradrenergic function and panic anxiety effects of yohimbine in health subjects and patients with agoraphobia and panic disorder. Arch Gen Psychiatry 41:751–763, 1984

Charney D, Heninger G, Jatlow P: Increased anxiogenic effects of caffeine in panic disorders. Arch Gen Psychiatry 42:233–243, 1985

Charney DS, Woods SW, Goodman WK, et al: Drug treatment of panic disorder: the comparative efficacy of imipramine, alprazolam, and trazodone. J Clin Psychiatry 47:580–586, 1986

Charney DS, Woods SW, Goodman WK, et al: Neurobiological mechanisms of panic anxiety: biochemical and behavioral correlates of yohimbine-induced panic attacks. Am J Psychiatry 144:1030–1036, 1987

Charney DS, Woods SW, Nagy LM, et al: Noradrenergic function of panic disorder. J Clin Psychiatry 51(12, suppl A):5–11, 1990

Chouinard G, Annable L, Fontaine R, et al: Alprazolam in the treatment of generalized anxiety and panic disorders: a double-blind placebo-controlled study. Psychopharmacology (Berlin) 77:229–233, 1982

Clark DM: A cognitive approach to panic. Behav Res Ther 24:461–470, 1986

Clark DM, Salkovskis PM, Chalkley AJ: Respiratory control as a treatment for panic attacks. J Behav Ther Exp Psychiatry 16:23–30, 1985

Clark DM, Salkovskis PM, Gelder MG, et al: Tests of a cognitive theory of panic, in: Panic and Phobias II. Edited by Hand I, Wittchen HU. New York, Springer-Verlag, 1988

Clark DM, Salkovskis PM, Hackmann A, et al: A comparison of cognitive therapy, applied relaxation and imipramine in the treatment of panic disorder. (submitted for publication)

Cohen ME, Badal DW, Kilpatrick A, et al: The high familial prevalence of neurocirculatory asthenia (anxiety neurosis, effort syndrome). Am J Hum Genet 3:126, 1951

Committee on the Review of Medicines: Systematic review of the benzodiazepines. Br Med J 1:910–912, 1980

Coryell W: Mortality of anxiety disorders, in Handbook of Anxiety, Vol 2: Classification, Biological Factors and Associated Disturbances. Edited by Noyes R Jr, Roth M, Burrows GD. Amsterdam, Netherlands, Elsevier, 1988, pp 311–320

Coryell W, Noyes R, Clancy J: Excess mortality in panic disorder: a comparison with primary unipolar depression. Arch Gen Psychiatry 39:701–703, 1982

Coryell W, Noyes R, House JD: Mortality among outpatients with panic disorder. Am J Psychiatry 143:508–510, 1986

Cowley DS, Roy-Byrne P: Psychosocial aspects. Psychiatric Annals 18(8):464–467, 1988

Craske M, Barlow D: A review of the relationship between panic and avoidance. Clinical Psychology Review 8(6):667–685, 1988

Cross-National Collaborative Panic Study: Drug treatment of panic disorder: comparative efficacy of alprazolam, imipramine, and placebo. Br J Psychiatry 160:191–202, 1992

Crowe RR: Family and twin studies of panic disorder and agoraphobia, in Handbook of Anxiety, Vol 1: Biological, Clinical and Cultural Perspectives. Edited by Roth M, Noyes R Jr, Burrows GD. Amsterdam, Netherlands, Elsevier, 1988, pp 101–114

Davidson JRT: Continuation treatment of panic disorder with high-potency benzodiazepines. J Clin Psychiatry 51:31–37, 1990 de la Fuente JR: Drug treatment of panic anxiety. Paper presented at the 141st annual meeting of the American Psychiatric Association, Montreal, Quebec, Canada, May 1988

Dunner DL, Ishiki D, Avery DH, et al: Effect of alprazolam and diazepam on anxiety and panic attacks in panic disorder: a controlled study. J Clin Psychiatry 47:458–460, 1986

Dupont RL: Thinking about stopping treatment for panic disorder. J Clin Psychiatry 51:38–45, 1990

Eaton WW, Kessler LG: Epidemiologic field methods in psychiatry: the NIMH Epidemiologic Catchment Area Program. Orlando, FL, Academic Press, 1985

Eaton WW, Holzer CE III, Von Korff M, et al: The design of the Epidemiologic Catchment Area surveys: the control and measurement of error. Arch Gen Psychiatry 41:942–948, 1984

Eaton WW, Dryman A, Weissman MM: Panic and phobia, in Psychiatric Disorders in America. Edited by Robins LN, Regier DA. New York, Free Press, 1990, pp 155–179

Edwards JG, Inman WHW, Pearce GL, et al: Prescription-event monitoring of 10895 patients treated with alprazolam. Br J Psychiatry 158:387–392, 1991

Escobar JI, Landbloom RP: Treatment of phobic neurosis with clomipramine: a controlled clinical trial. Curr Ther Res 20:680–685, 1976

Faravelli C, Pallanti S: Recent life events and panic disorder. Am J Psychiatry146:622–626, 1989

Faravelli C, Webb T, Ambonetti A, et al: Prevalence of traumatic early life events in 31 agoraphobic patients with panic attacks. Am J Psychiatry 142(12):1493–1494, 1985

Fawcett J: Targeting treatment in patients with mixed symptoms of anxiety and depression. J Clin Psychiatry 51:40–43, 1990

Fontaine R, Chouinard G, Annable K: Rebound anxiety in anxious patients after abrupt withdrawal of benzodiazepine treatment. Am J Psychiatry 141:848–852, 1984

Fossey MD, Lydiard RB: Anxiety and the gastrointestinal system. Psychiatr Med 8(3):175–186, 1990

Fyer AJ, Sandberg D: Pharmacologic treatment of panic disorder, in Review of Psychiatry, Vol 7. Edited by Hales RE, Frances AJ. Washington, DC, American Psychiatric Press, 1988

Gelder MG, Clark DM, Salkovskis P: Psychological treatment for panic disorder. J Psychiatr Res (in press)

Gelenberg AJ: Quality of life with clozapine. Biological Therapies in Psychiatry 14(3):11, 1991

Gittelman R, Klein DF: Relationship between separation anxiety panic and agoraphobic disorders. Psychopathology 17:15–65, 1984

Gorman JM, Liebowitz MR, Fyer, AJ, et al: Possible respiratory abnormalities in panic disorder. Psychopharmacol Bull 22:792–796, 1986

Gorman JM, Liebowitz MR, Fyer AJ, et al: An open trial of fluoxetine in the treatment of panic attacks. J Clin Psychopharmacol 7:329–332, 1987

Gorman JM, Battista D, Goetz RR, et al: A comparison of sodium bicarbonate and sodium lactate infusion in the induction of panic attacks. Arch Gen Psychiatry 46:145–150, 1989

Grandi S, Fava GA, Luria E: Sintomi ipocondriaci nell'agorafobia [Hypochondriacal symptoms in agoraphobia]. 11th National Congress of the Italian Society of Psychosomatic Medicine (1987, Messina, Italy). Medicina Psicosomatica 33(1):19–27, 1988

Gray J: A theory of anxiety: the role of the limbic system. Encephale 9(4, suppl 2):161B–166B, 1983

Greden JF: Anxiety or caffeinism: a diagnosis dilemma. Am J Psychiatry 131:1089–1092, 1974

Griffiths RR, Bigelow GE, Liebsin I, et al: Drug preference in humans: double-blind choice comparison of pentobarbital, diazepam, and placebo J Pharmacol Exp Ther 215:649–661, 1980

Griffiths RR, McLeod DR, Bigelow GE, et al: Relative abuse liability of diazepam and oxazepam: behavioral and subjective dose effects. Psychopharmacology (Berlin) 84:147–154, 1983

Hamilton M: The assessment of anxiety states by rating. Br J Med Psychol 32:50–55, 1959

Hand I, Wittchen HU (eds): Panic and Phobias. Berlin, Springer-Verlag, 1986

Harrison M, Busto U, Naranjo CA, et al: Diazepam tapering in detoxification for high-dose benzodiazepine abuse. Clin Pharmacol Ther 36:527–533, 1986

Heinrichs DW, Hanlon ET, Carpenter WT Jr: The Quality of Life Scale: an instrument for rating the schizophrenic deficit syndrome. Schizophr Bull 10:388–398, 1984

Himle JA, Crystal D, Curtis GC, et al: Mode of onset of simple phobia subtypes: further evidence of heterogeneity. Psychiatry Res 36(1):37–43, 1991

Hollander E, Liebowitz MR, Gorman JM, et al: Cortisol and sodium lactate-induced panic. Arch Gen Psychiatry 46:135–140, 1989

Hollander E, Hatterer J, Klein DF: Antidepressants for the treatment of panic and agoraphobia, in Handbook of Anxiety, Vol 4: Treatment of Anxiety. Edited by Noyes R Jr, Roth M, Burrows GD. Amsterdam, Netherlands, Elsevier, 1990, pp 207–231

Hwu HG, Yeh EK, Chang LY: Prevalence of psychiatric disorders in Taiwan defined by the Chinese diagnostic interview schedule. Acta Psychiatr Scand 79(2):136–147, 1989

Johnston DG, Troyer IE, Whitsett SF: Clomipramine treatment of agoraphobic women. Arch Gen Psychiatry 45:453–459, 1988

Judd FK, Burrows GD, Marriott PF, et al: A short-term open clinical trial of clobazam in the treatment of patients with panic attacks. Int Clin Psychopharmacol 4:285–294, 1989

Kabat-Zinn J, Massion AO, Kristseller J, et al: Effectiveness of a meditation-based stress reduction program in the treatment of anxiety disorders. Am J Psychiatry 149:936–943, 1992

Kagan J, Reznick JS, Snidman N, et al: Origins of panic disorder, in Neurobiology of Anxiety. Edited by Ballenger JC. New York, Alan R Liss, 1990

Kahn RS, Westenberg HGM, Verhoeven WMA, et al: Effect of serotonin precursors and uptake inhibitor in anxiety disorders: a double-blind comparison of 5-hydroxytryptophan, clomipramine and placebo. Int Clin Psychopharmacol 2:21–32, 1987

Karabanow O: Double-blind controlled study in phobias and obsessions. J Int Med Res 5:42–48, 1977

Katschnig H, Pakesch G, Loimer N, et al: Panic attacks and depressive symptoms in a population survey in Vienna. Pharmacopsychiatry 21:62, 1988

Katschnig H, Stolk JM, Klerman GL, et al: Long-term follow-up of panic disorder, I: clinical outcomes of a large group of patients participating in an international multicenter clinical drug trial. (submitted for publication)

Keller MB: The natural history of panic disorder. Paper presented at the Annual Meeting of the American Psychiatric Association. New Orleans, LA, May 1991

Keller MB, Hanks DL: Course and outcome in panic disorder. Prog Neuropsychopharmcol Biol Psychiatry (in press)

Klein DF, Rabkin JG (eds): Anxiety: New Research and Changing Concepts. New York, Raven, 1981

Klerman GL: Treatments for panic disorder. J Clin Psychiatry 53 (suppl):14–19, 1992

Klerman GL, Lavori P: Drug treatment of panic disorder: comparative efficacy of alprazolam, imipramine and placebo. Br J Psychiatry (in press)

Klerman GL, Ballenger JC, Burrows GD, et al: The efficacy of alprazolam in panic disorder and agoraphobia: a critique of recent reports (letter). Arch Gen Psychiatry 46: 670–672, 1989

Lader MH: Benzodiazepine withdrawal, in Handbook of Anxiety, Vol 4: Treatment of Anxiety. Edited by Noyes R Jr, Roth M, Burrows GD. Amsterdam, Netherlands, Elsevier, 1990, pp 57–71

Lader MH, Lawson C: Sleep studies and rebound insomnia: methodological problems, laboratory findings, and clinical implications. Clin Neuropharmacol 10:291–312, 1987

Laughren TP, Battey YW, Greenblatt DJ: Chronic diazepam treatment in psychiatric outpatients. J Clin Psychiatry 4:461–462, 1982a

Laughren TP, Battey YW, Greenblatt DJ, et al: A controlled trial of diazepam withdrawal in chronically anxious outpatients. Acta Psychiatr Scand 65:171–179, 1982b

Lesser IM: Panic disorder and depression: co-occurrence and treatment, in Clinical Aspects of Panic Disorder. Edited by Ballenger J. New York, Wiley-Liss, 1980

Lesser IM: The relationship between panic disorder and depression. J Anxiety Disord 2:3–15, 1988

Lesser IM: Diagnostic considerations in panic disorders, in Handbook of Phobia Therapy. Edited by Lindemann C. Northvale, NJ, Jason Aronson, 1989, pp 17–38

Lesser IM, Rubin RT: Diagnostic considerations in panic disorders. J Clin Psychiatry 47:4–10, 1986

Lesser IM, Rubin RT, Lydiard RB, et al: Past and current thyroid function in patients with panic disorder. J Clin Psychiatry 48:473–476, 1987

Levy AB: Delirium and seizures due to abrupt alprazolam withdrawal: case report. J Clin Psychiatry 45:38–39, 1984

Liebowitz MR, Fyer AJ, Gorman JM, et al: Alprazolam in the treatment of panic disorders. J Clin Psychopharmacol 6:13–20, 1986a

Liebowitz MR, Fyer AJ, Gorman J, et al: Recent developments in the understanding and pharamacotherapy of panic attacks. Psychopharmacol Bull 22:792–796, 1986b

Litovitz TL, Schmitz Bf, Bailey KM: 1989 Annual report of the American Association of Poison Control Centers National Data Collection System. Am J Emerg Med 394–430, 1990

Lydiard RB, Roy-Byrne PP, Ballenger JC: Recent advances in the psychopharmacological treatment of anxiety disorders. Hosp Community Psychiatry 39:1157–1165, 1988

Majewska MD, Harrison NL, Schwartz RD, et al: Steroid hormone metabolites are barbituate-like modulators of the GABA receptor. Science 232:1004–1007, 1986

Marks IM: Are there anticompulsive or antiphobic drugs? review of the evidence. Br J Psychiatry 143:338–347, 1983

Marks IM: Fears, Phobias and Rituals. New York, Oxford University Press, 1987

Marks IM, Marks M: Exposure treatment of agoraphobia/panic, in Handbook of Anxiety, Vol 4: Treatment of Anxiety. Edited by Noyes R Jr, Roth M, Burrows GD. Amsterdam, Netherlands, Elsevier, 1990, pp 293–310

Marks IM, Swinson RP: Behavioral and/or drug therapy, in Handbook of Anxiety, Vol 5. Edited by Burrows G, Roth M, Noyes R. Amsterdam, Netherlands, Elsevier, 1992, pp 255–268

Mavissakalian M, Dealy R: Pharmacological treatment of agoraphobia: imipramine vs. imipramine with programmed practice. Br J Psychiatry 143:348–355, 1985

McTavish D, Benfield P: Clomipramine: an overview of its pharmacological properties and a review of its therapeutic use in obsessive compulsive disorder and panic disorder. Drugs 39:136–153, 1990

Mellinger GD, Balter MB: Prevalence and patterns of use of psychotherapeutic drugs: results from a 1979 national survey of American adults, in Epidemiological Impact of Psychotropic Drugs: Proceedings of the International

Seminar on the Impact of Psychotropic Drugs. Edited by Totnoni G, Bellantuano C, Lader M. Amsterdam, Netherlands, North Holland Publishing Company, 1981, pp 117–135

Mellinger GD, Balter MB, Manheimer DI, et al: Psychic distress, life crisis, and use of psychotherapeutic medications: national household survey data. Arch Gen Psychiatry 35:1045–1052, 1978

Mellinger GD, Balter MB, Uhlenhuth EH, et al: Evaluating a household survey measure of psychic distress. Psychol Med 13:607–621, 1983

Mellinger GD, Balter MB, Uhlenhuth EH: Anti-anxiety agents: duration of use and characteristics of users in the USA. Curr Med Res Opin 8(suppl 4):21–36, 1984

Mellinger GD, Balter MB, Uhlenhuth EH: Insomnia and its treatment. Arch Gen Psychiatry 42:225–232, 1985

Mellman TA, Uhde TW: Withdrawal syndrome with gradual tapering of alprazolam. Am J Psychiatry 143:1464–1466, 1986

Modigh K: Antidepressant drugs in anxiety disorders. Acta Psychiatr Scand 76:57–71, 1987

Modigh K, Westberg P, Eriksson E: Superiority of clomipramine over imipramine in the treatment of panic disorder: a placebo-controlled trial. Paper presented at the 17th Congress of Collegium International Neuro-Psychopharmacologicum, Kyoto, Japan, September 1990

Moras K, Craske MG, Barlow DH: Behavioral and cognitive therapies for panic disorder, in Handbook of Anxiety, Vol 4: Treatment of Anxiety. Edited by Noyes R Jr, Roth N, Burrows GD. Amsterdam, Netherlands, Elsevier, 1990, pp 311–325

Mountjoy CQ, Roth M, Garside RF, et al: A clinical trial of phenelzine in anxiety, depression and phobic neurosis. Br J Psychiatry 131:486–492, 1977

Mukerji V, Beitman B, Alpert M, et al: Panic disorder: a frequent occurrence in patients with chest pain and normal coronary arteries. Angiology 38(3):236–240, 1987

Noyes R Jr: The natural history of anxiety disorders, in Handbook of Anxiety, Vol 1: Biological, Clinical and Cultural Perspectives. Edited by Roth M, Noyes R Jr, Burrows GD. Amsterdam, Netherlands, Elsevier, 1988, pp 115–133

Noyes R Jr, Perry P: Maintenance treatment with antidepresssants in panic disorder. J Clin Psychiatry 51:24–30, 1990

Noyes R Jr, Clancy J, Crowe RR, et al: The familial prevalence of anxiety neurosis. Arch Gen Psychiatry 39:1057–1059, 1978

Noyes R, Clancy J, Hoenck PR, et al: The prognosis of anxiety neurosis. Arch Gen Psychiatry 37:173–178, 1980

Noyes R, Anderson DJ, Clancy J, et al: Diazepam and propranolol in panic disorder and agoraphobia. Arch Gen Psychiatry 41:287–292, 1984

Noyes R Jr, Clancy J, Coryell WH, et al: A withdrawal syndrome after abrupt discontinuation of alprazolam. Am J Psychiatry 142:114–116, 1985

Noyes R, Crowe RR, Harris EL, et al: Relationship between panic disorder and agoraphobia. Arch Gen Psychiatry 43:227–232, 1986

Noyes R Jr, Clancy J, Garvey MJ, et al: Is agoraphobia a variant of panic disorder or a separate illness? J Anxiety Disorders 1:3–13, 1987a

Noyes R, Clarkson C, Crowe R, et al: A family study of generalized anxiety disorder. Am J Psychiatry 144:1019–1024, 1987b

Noyes R Jr, Dupont RL, Pecknold JC, et al: Alprazolam in panic disorder and agoraphobia: results from a multicenter trial, II: patient acceptance, side effects, and safety. Arch Gen Psychiatry 45:423–428, 1988

Noyes R Jr, Roth M, Burrows GD: Handbook of Anxiety. Amsterdam, Netherlands, Elsevier, 1990

Nutt DJ, Glue P, Lawson C, et al: Flumazenil provocation of panic attacks. Arch Gen Psychiatry 47:917–925, 1990

Olfson M, Klerman GL: The treatment of depression: prescribing practices of primary care physicians and psychiatrists. J Fam Pract 35(6):627–635, 1992

Öst L, Hugdahl K: Acquisition of agoraphobia, mode of onset and anxiety response pattern. Behav Res Ther 21(6):623–631, 1983

O'Sullivan G, Marks I: Long-term outcome of phobic and obsessive-compulsive disorders after treatment, in Handbook of Anxiety, Vol 4: Treatment of Anxiety. Edited by Noyes R Jr, Roth M, Burrows GD. Amsterdam, Netherlands, Elsevier, 1990, pp 87–108

Parry HJ, Balter MB, Mellinger GD, et al: National patterns of psychotherapeutic drug use. Arch Gen Psychiatry 28:769–783, 1973

Pauls DL, Noyes R Jr, Crowe RR: Familial prevalence in second-degree relatives of patients with anxiety neurosis. J Affect Disord 1:279–285, 1979

Petursson H, Lader M: Withdrawal from long-term benzodiazepine treatment. BMJ 283:643–645, 1981

Pevnick JS, Jasinski DR, Haertzen CA: Abrupt withdrawal from therapeutically administered diazepam. Arch Gen Psychiatry 35:995–998, 1978

Pichot P: History of the treatment of anxiety, in Handbook of Anxiety, Vol 4: Treatment of Anxiety. Edited by Noyes R Jr, Roth M, Burrows GD. Amsterdam, Netherlands, Elsevier, 1990, pp 3–25

Pollack MH, Tesar GE, Rosenbaum JF, et al: Clonazepam in the treatment of panic disorder and agoraphobia: a one-year follow-up. J Clin Psychopharmacol 6:302–304, 1986

Pollack MH, Rosenbaum JF, Tesar G, et al: Clonazepam in the treatment of panic disorder and agoraphobia. Psychopharmacol Bull 23:141–144, 1987

Pollack MH, Otto MW, Rosenbaum JF, et al: Longitudinal course of panic disorder: findings from the Massachusetts General Hospital Naturalistic Study. J Clin Psychiatry 51:12–16, 1990

Reiman EM: Positron emission tomography in the study of panic disorder and anticipatory anxiety, in Handbook of Anxiety, Vol 3. Edited by Burrows M, Roth M, Noyes R Jr. Amsterdam, Netherlands, Elsevier, 1991, pp 289–306

Reiman EM, Raichle ME, Robins E, et al: Neuroanatomical correlates of a lactate-induced panic attack. Arch Gen Psychiatry 46:493–500, 1989

Rickels K: Benzodiazepines: use and misuse, in Anxiety: New Research and Changing Concepts. Edited by Klein DF, Rabkin JG. New York, Raven, 1981, pp 1–26

Rickels K: Antianxiety therapy: potential value of long-term treatment. J Clin Psychiatry 48(suppl):7–11, 1987

Rickels K, Schweizer EE: Benzodiazepines for the treatment of panic attacks: a new look. Psychopharmacol Bull 2:93–99, 1986

Rickels K, Case WG, Schweizer EE, et al: Low-dose dependence in chronic benzodiazepine users: a preliminary report on 119 patients. Psychopharmacol Bull 22:407–415, 1986

Rickels K, Schweitzer E, Case WG, et al: Long-term therapeutic use of benzodiazepines, I: effects of abrupt discontinuation. Arch Gen Psychiatry 47:899–907, 1990

Rifkin A, Quitkin F, Klein DS: Withdrawal reaction to diazepam. JAMA 236:2172–2173, 1976

Rifkin A, Pecknold JC, Swinson RP, et al: Sequence of improvement in agoraphobia with panic attacks. J Psychiatr Res 24:1–8, 1990

Robins LN, Helzer JE, Weissman MM, et al: Lifetime prevalence of specific psychiatric disorders in three sites. Arch Gen Psychiatry 41:949–958, 1984

Rosenbaum JF, Biederman J, Gersten J, et al: Behavioral inhibition in children of parents with panic disorder and agoraphobia: a controlled study. Arch Gen Psychiatry 45:463–470, 1988

Roth M, Myers DH: Anxiety neuroses and phobic states: diagnosis and management. Br Med J 1:559–562, 1969

Roth M, Gurney C, Garside RF, et al: Studies in the classification of affective disorders: the relationship between anxiety states and depressive illnesses. Br J Psychiatry 121:147–162, 1972

Roy-Byrne P, Geraci M, Uhde T: Life events and course of illness in patients with panic disorder. Am J Psychiatry 143(8): 1033–1035, 1986

Rubin RT, Lesser IM: Psychoneuroendocrinological aspects of depression, anxiety, and related disorders. Psychiatria Fennica Supplementum 17:9–17, 1986

Schapira K, Roth M, Kerr TA, et al: The prognosis of affective disorders: the differentiation of anxiety states from depressive illnesses. Br J Psychiatry 121:175–183, 1972

Schweitzer E, Rickels K, Case WG, et al: Long-term therapeutic use of benzodiazepines, II: effects of gradual taper. Arch Gen Psychiatry 47:908–915, 1990

Senay EC: Addictive behaviors and benzodiazepines, 1: abuse liability and physical dependence. Adv Alcohol Subst Abuse 8:107–124, 1989

Sheehan DV: Benzodiazepines in panic disorder and agoraphobia. J Affect Disord 13:169–181, 1987

Sheehan DV, Raj BA: Benzodiazepine treatment of panic disorder, in Handbook of Anxiety, Vol 4: Treatment of Anxiety. Edited by Noyes R Jr, Roth M, Burrows GD. Amsterdam, Netherlands, Elsevier, 1990, pp 169–206

Sheehan DV, Claycomb JB, Surman OS: The relative efficacy of phenelzine, imipramine, alprazolam, and placebo in the treatment of panic attacks and agoraphobia. Paper presented at the meeting on Biology and Panic Disorders, Boston, MA, November 1983

Sheehan DV, Claycomb JB, Surman OS, et al: Comparison of phenelzine, imipramine, alprazolam, and placebo in the treatment of panic attacks and agoraphobia. Paper presented at the annual meeting of the American Psychiatric Association Annual Meeting, Los Angeles, CA, May 1984

Siber A: Panic attacks facilitating recall and mastery: implications for psychoanalytic technique. J Am Psychoanal Assoc 37(2):337–364, 1989

Smith DE, Wesson DR, Landry M: The pharmacology of benzodiazepine addiction. Family Practice Recertification 11(suppl):94–106, 1989

Solyom C, Solyom L, LaPierre Y, et al: Phenelzine and exposure in the treatment of phobias. J Biol Psychiatry 16:239–248, 1981

Spitzer RL, Williams J: Instructional Manual for the Structured Clinical Interview for DSM-III (SCID). New York, New York Biomedical Research Department, New York State Psychiatric Institute, 1985

Stone MH: Psychotherapy for the treatment of anxiety disorders, in Handbook of Anxiety, Vol 4: Treatment of Anxiety. Edited by Noyes R Jr, Roth M, Burrows GD. Amsterdam, Netherlands, Elsevier, 1990, pp 389–404

Sullivan MD, Katon W, Roy-Byrne P: Treatment of anxiety in primary care, in Handbook of Anxiety, Vol 4: Treatment of Anxiety. Edited by Noyes R Jr, Roth M, Burrows GD. Amsterdam, Netherlands, Elsevier, 1990, pp 427–448

Torgersen S: Genetics of anxiety and its clinical implications, in Handbook of Anxiety, Vol 3: The Neurobiology of Anxiety. Edited by Burrows GD, Roth M, Noyes R Jr. New York, Elsevier, 1991, pp 381–406

Tuma AH, Maser JD: Anxiety and the Anxiety Disorders. Hillsdale, NJ, Erlbaum, 1985

Tyrer P: Neurosis divisible. Lancet 1:685–688, 1984

Tyrer P: Classification of anxiety disorders. Journal of Anxiety Disorders 11:991–994, 1986

Tyrer P, Shawcross C: Monoamine oxidase inhibitors in anxiety disorders. J Psychiatr Res 22 (suppl 1): 87–98, 1988

Vollrath M, Koch R, Angst J: The Zurich study. panic disorder and sporadic panic: symptoms, diagnosis, prevalence, and overlap with depression. Psychiatry Neurol Sci 239:221–230, 1990

Weissman MM: Panic and generalized anxiety: are they separate disorders? J Psychiatr Res 24(suppl 2):157–162, 1990

Weissman MM, Myers JK, Harding PS: Psychiatric disorders in a United States urban community: 1975–76. Am J Psychiatry 135:459–462, 1978

Wheeler ED, White PD, Reed E, et al: Familial incidence of neurocirculatory asthenia ("anxiety neurosis," "effort syndrome"). J Clin Invest 27:562, 1948

Winokur A, Rickels K, Greenblatt DJ, et al: Withdrawal reaction from long-term, low-dosage administration of diazepam. Arch Gen Psychiatry 37:101–105, 1980

Wittchen HU: Epidemiology of panic attacks and panic disorder, in Panic and Phobias. Edited by Hand I, Wittchen HU. New York, Springer-Verlag, 1986, pp 18–27

Zitrin CM, Klein DF, Woerner MG: Behavior therapy, supportive psychotherapy, imipramine and phobias. Arch Gen Psychiatry 35:307–316, 1978

Index

Page numbers printed in **boldface** type refer to tables or figures.

Abnormal endogenous ligand
theory, 51
Activation reactions
with benzodiazepines, 76
with tricyclic antidepressants, 67,
68, 69, 70
Addictive potential, of
benzodiazepines, 77
Adjunctive treatment, benzodiazepine withdrawal and, 80–81
Age at onset, as risk factor, 22
Agoraphobia. *See also* Comorbid
panic disorder, agoraphobia and
clinical description of, 58
without panic attacks, 26
parental child-rearing behavior
and, 46
treatment of
exposure-based therapy in, 91
imipramine combined with
psychological therapy in,
103–104
long-term psychological
treatment and, 98
Alcohol, withdrawal from, 17
Alcoholism
comorbidity with, 26, 28–29
prevalence of, 37
Alpha2-adrenoreceptor receptors, as
markers, 48
3 Alpha, 5 alpha-tetrahydroxycorticosterone, hypnotic-
anxiolytic effect produced by, 51
3 Alpha-hydroxy-5 alpha-dihydroprogesterone, hypnotic-
anxiolytic effect produced by, 51
Alphaxalone, reduction of anxiety
behavior by, 51

Alprazolam, 65, 71, **71,** 87–89
as antipanic medication, **64**
comparative studies of, 84
diazepam and, 76
imipramine and, 73–75, **74, 75**
lorazepam and, 76
psychological treatment and,
100–101
in depression, 84
discontinuation of, 78, 87
dosage of, **71,** 72, 87
maintenance, 70
efficacy of, 75–76
pharmacodynamic explanation
of, 75
pharmacokinetic explanation of,
75–76
long-term treatment with, 86
rebound with, 79
Amphetamines, precipitation of
anxiety attacks by, 17
Amygdaloid nuclei, anxiety-arousal
states and, 48
Anger, toleration of, 54–55
Angiograms, 19, 20
Animal models, of anxiety and
arousal states, 48
Anticholinergic effects, of tricyclic
antidepressants, 69
Anticipatory anxiety, 13
learning theory of, 43
treatment of, 70
Antidepressants. *See also* Tricyclic
antidepressants
rates of use of, 110
Antipanic medications, **64,** 64–65.
*See also specific drugs and drug
classes*

Anxiety
  animal models of, 48
  anticipatory, 13
    learning theory of, 43
    treatment of, 70
  increase in
    with benzodiazepines, 76
    with tricyclic antidepressants,
      67, 68, 69, 70
  limited symptom attacks and, 7
  panic, 6–7
    clinical manifestations of, 7, **8, 9**
    symptoms of, 7, **7**
  separation, etiology of panic
    disorder and, 45
  signal, 42
Anxiety attacks, precipitation by
  drugs of abuse, 17
Anxiety disorders
  comorbidity with, 13–14, 26–27
  differentiation of panic disorder
    from, 59
  separation of panic disorder and,
    23
Anxiety neurosis, 4–5
  Freud's use of, 4, 42
Anxiolytics. *See also*
    Benzodiazepine(s); *specific drugs*
  in comorbid panic disorder with
    agoraphobia, 111
  psychological therapy combined
    with, 105
  rates of use of, 109
  serotonin turnover and, 50
Applied relaxation (AR), 92
  in agoraphobia, 98
  progressive muscle relaxation
    compared with, 93
  psychopharmacological treatment
    compared with, 101–102
Arousal states
  animal models of, 48
  worsening of chronic medical
    illness by, 20
Assessment, 14–15, **15**
Asthma, hospitalizations for, 20
Ataxia, with benzodiazepines, 76

Autonomic arousal
  animal models of, 48
  worsening of chronic medical
    illness by, 20
Avoidance behavior. *See* Phobic
    avoidance

Behavioral inhibition, childhood,
    etiology of panic disorder and,
    45–46
Behavior theories, of etiology of
    panic disorder, 43–44
Behavior therapy. *See*
    Cognitive-behavioral treatment
Benzodiazepine(s), 62, 64, **71,** 71–81,
    87–89, 114–115. *See also*
    specific drugs
  abuse potential of, 76–77
  as antipanic medications, **64**
  clinical discontinuation reactions
    and, 78, **79**
  in comorbid panic disorder
    with agoraphobia, 111
    with substance abuse, 77
  comparative studies of, 84, **85**
  dependence on, 77–78
  discontinuation of, 115
  effectiveness in panic disorder, 27
  general considerations with, **71,**
    71–73
  patterns of use of, 110
  rates of use of, 109
  rebound with, 79, **80**
  side effects of, 76
  with tricyclic antidepressants, 70
  withdrawal from, factors
    influencing, 79–81, **81**
Benzodiazepine gamma-aminobutyric
    acid receptor theory, 50–51
Benzodiazepines
  relapse following treatment with,
    79, **80,** 87
  withdrawal from, 76, 78, **79,** 115
Beta-adrenergic blocking agents, in
    mitral valve prolapse,
    differential diagnosis of panic
    disorder and, 17

Biological markers, 48
Blood flow, cerebral, 49
Blood pressure, changes in, with
    tricyclic antidepressants, 69, 88
Bodily sensations, misinterpretation
    of, 44–45
    cognitive-behavioral treatment
        and, 93, 95
Brain imaging studies, 48–49
Brain structures
    anxiety-arousal states and, 48
    changes in, 52–53
Breathing retraining, 93, 94
    comparative outcome studies of, 98
Buspirone, 27
    anxiolytic action of, 50
BZ anxiolytics, serotonin turnover
    and, 50
BZ receptor, dysfunction in, 53
BZ receptor-GABA-A-Cl⁻-ionophore
    complex, regulation of, 50–51

Caffeine, anxiogenic effects of, 17
Caffeine provocation, 5, 47
    validity of panic disorder as
        nosological entity and, 58
Carbon dioxide provocation, 5, 47
    validity of panic disorder as
        nosological entity and, 58
Cardiac conduction times, tricyclic
    antidepressants and, 69
"Cardiac neuroses," 4
Cardiomyopathy, comorbidity with,
    34
Cardiovascular disease
    comorbidity with, 34
    imipramine and, 69
    mortality and, 35
    risk for stroke in patients with
        panic disorder, 30
Cerebral blood flow, 49
Challenge studies, 5, 47–48, 50
Childhood behavioral inhibition,
    etiology of panic disorder and,
    45–46
Child-rearing, etiology of panic
    disorder and, 46

Chlorazepate, 71, **71,** 73
    dosage of, **71**
Chlordiazepoxide, 71, **71**
    dosage of, **71**
m-Chloro-phenyl-piperazine
    provocation, 50
Cholecystokinin provocation, 47
Chronic fatigue syndrome, 20
Clinical course, 30–32, **32, 33**
Clinical features, 8–9, 13–14
Clomipramine, 68
    comparative studies of, 84
    fluvoxamine and, 81–82
    dosage of, 68, 70
    side effects of, 68, 69, 70
Clonazepam, 71, **71,** 76
    as antipanic medication, **64**
    dosage of, **71**
Clonidine, growth hormone
    response to, in depression and
    panic disorder, 27
Clonidine provocation, 50
Cocaine
    precipitation of anxiety attacks
        by, 17
    stimulation of brain receptors
        associated with anxiety by, 17
Cognitive-behavioral treatment, 44,
    93–98
    in clinical practice, 112
    comparative outcome studies of,
        95–98, 98
    antidepressants and, 105
    anxiolytics and, 105
    imipramine and, 103–104
    psychopharmacological
        treatment and, 101–102
Cognitive impairment, with
    benzodiazepines, 76
Cognitive restructuring (CR), 93
    comparative outcome studies of,
        97–98
    with interoceptive exposure,
        comparative outcome studies
        of, 96
Cognitive theory, of etiology of panic
    disorder, 44–45

Communication skills training, 92
Community, prescription and use of
     antipanic medications in. *See*
     Psychopharmacological
     treatment, community patterns
     of prescription and use of
     antipanic medications and
Comorbid panic disorder, 20, 21, 32
  with agoraphobia, 13, 25–26
     alcoholism and, 28
     American and European views
          of, 25, 26
     clomipramine in, 68
     cognitive-behavioral treatment
          in, 94–95, 96
     comparative outcome studies of
          treatments in, 97–98, 99
     imipramine combined with
          psychological therapy in,
          104–105
     personality characteristics and,
          54
     personality disorders and, 28
     sequence of panic attacks in, 25
     supportive therapy in, 96
     treatment of, 111
  with alcoholism, 26, 28–29
  with anxiety disorders, 13–14,
     26–27
  with depression, 27–28
     familial relationship between
          panic disorder and, 41
     impairment in, 32
     psychopharmacological treat-
          ment response and, 83–84
  with medical illness, 29–30, 34–35
     mortality and, 34–35
  with personality disorders, 28
  with substance abuse, 26, 28–29
     benzodiazepines in treatment
          of, 77
Conditioning, etiology of panic
     disorder and, 43–44
Conduction times, tricyclic
     antidepressants and, 69
Convulsive disorders, panic disorder
     as variant of, 52

Criticism, parental, etiology of panic
     disorder and, 46
Cross-cultural studies, 23–24
Cross-National Collaborative Panic
     Study (CNCPS), 38, 60, 72,
     73–75, **74, 75,** 83–84, 86
Cross-national studies, 23–24, 38,
     60, 72, 73–75, **74, 75,** 83–84, 86
Culture-specific syndromes, 23

Death, 34–36
  cardiovascular disease and, 35
  suicide and, 34, 35–36
Dependence
  on benzodiazepines, 77–78
  therapeutic levels of, 62
Depersonalization disorder,
     differential diagnosis of panic
     disorder and, 16
Depression
  atypical, 16
  comorbidity with. *See* Comorbid
     panic disorder, with
     depression
  differential diagnosis of panic
     disorder and, 15–16
  familial relationship between
     panic disorder and, 41
  suicide risk and, 35
Desipramine, 67
  as antipanic medication, **64**
  dosage of, 67
  side effects of, 69
Developmental theories, of etiology
     of panic disorder, 45–46
Diagnosis, 8–9
  benzodiazepine withdrawal and,
     80
  delays in, problems associated
     with, 20–21
  diagnostic criteria and
     DSM-III-R, **8**
     ICD-10, 9
     operational, 5–6
  diagnostic validity and. *See*
     Validity as nosological entity
  differential, 15–17

medical disorders and, **16,** 16–17
psychiatric disorders and, 15, **16**
DSM and ICD and, 10–12, **11, 12**
misdiagnosis of panic disorder
and, 18–21
structured interviews for, 6
*Diagnostic and Statistical Manual
of Mental Disorders* (DSM), 1, 57
Third Edition, Revised
(DSM-III-R), 10, **11,** 11–12, 24
diagnostic criteria for panic
disorder and, **8**
Third Edition (DSM-III), 6, 10, **11,**
11–12, 24
Diagnostic Interview Schedule, 59
Diazepam, 71, **71,** 73
alprazolam compared with, 76
discontinuation of, 78
dosage of, **71,** 72, 76
patterns of use of, 110
rebound with, 79
with tricyclic antidepressants, 70
Diazepam binding inhibitor, 51
Differential diagnosis, 15–17
medical disorders and, **16,** 16–17
psychiatric disorders and, 15, **16**
Disinhibition phenomena
with benzodiazepines, 76
with tricyclic antidepressants, 67,
68, 69, 70
Dizziness, 20
Dopamine, release of, cocaine and, 17
Drug abuse. *See* Alcoholism;
Substance abuse
Drug therapy. *See*
Psychopharmacological
treatment; *specific drugs and
drug classes*

Economic disability, 38
Education, in clinical practice, 112
Egna Minnen Betraffande
Uppfostran (My Memories of
Upbringing [questionnaire]), 46
Electroencephalography (EEG), 52
tricyclic antidepressants and, 70
Emergency medical services, 20

Employment, 38
Epidemiologic Catchment Area
(ECA) study, 18, 21, 24–25, 30,
37, 38
Epidemiology, 21–24
cross-national and cross-cultural
considerations and, 23–24
pharmacoepidemiology and. *See*
Psychopharmacological treatment, community patterns of
prescription and use of
antipanic medications and
prevalence of alcoholism and, 37
prevalence of panic disorder and,
18, 21–22
delimitation from other
disorders and, 59
risk factors and, 22
family history as, 22–23
Etiology, 39–46
developmental theories of, 45–46
childhood behavioral inhibition
and, 45–46
childhood separation anxiety
and, 45
parental child-rearing attitudes
and behavior and, 46
genetics and familial factors in,
40–41
psychological theories of, 42–45
cognitive theory of, 44–45
learning and behavior theories
of, 43–44
psychodynamic and
psychoanalytic theories of,
42–43
Exposure-based therapy, 90–92, 93
in agoraphobia, 98
in clinical practice, 112
comparative outcome studies of,
97–98
cognitive restructuring and, 96
psychopharmacological
treatment and, 102–103
imipramine combined with,
104–105, 106, 107
including spouse in, 91–92, 99

Familial factors
    etiology of panic disorder and, 40
    as risk factor, 22–23
    validity of panic disorder as
        nosological entity and, 60
Fatigue, chronic, 20
Fears, developmentally significant,
    Freud's view of, 42
Flumazenil provocation, 47
Fluoxetine, 115
    side effects of, 69
Flurazepam, 71, **71**
    dosage of, **71**
Fluvoxamine, 81
    clomipramine compared with,
        81–82
Follow-up, 31–32, **32, 33**
Follow-up studies, validity of panic
    disorder as nosological entity
    and, 60
Fright disorders, 23–24

Gamma-aminobutyric acid. *See also*
    BZ receptor-GABA-A-Cl⁻-
    ionophore complex
    inhibitory effect of, 53
Gastrointestinal symptoms, 34
Gender
    comorbid anxiety disorder and,
        agoraphobia and alcoholism
        and, 29
    as risk factor, 22
Generalized anxiety disorder (GAD)
    comorbidity with, 26–27
    differentiation of panic disorder
        from, 59
Genetic linkage studies, 23
Genetics. *See also* Familial factors;
    Twin studies
    behavioral inhibition and, etiology
        of panic disorder and, 46
    etiology of panic disorder and, 40
Graduated exposure (GE), compara-
    tive outcome studies of, 97–98
Growth hormone response, to
    clonidine, in depression and
    panic disorder, 27

Halazepam, 71, **71**
    dosage of, **71**
Hallucinogens, precipitation of
    anxiety attacks by, 17
Harvard Anxiety Research Program
    (HARP), 28–29, 38, 60
Headaches, migraine, 20
Health care utilization, 37
Heart rate, changes in, with
    tricyclic antidepressants, 88
Help-seeking, 13, 18–19, 34
Hippocampus
    anxiety-arousal states and, 48
    blood flow in, 49
Hospitalization, 20
Hypercortisolemia, in depression
    and panic disorder, 27–28
Hyperventilation syndrome,
    clomipramine in, 68
Hypotension, orthostatic, with
    tricyclic antidepressants, 69
Hypothalamus, 52

Imipramine, 63, 65, 66–67
    as antipanic medication, **64**
    comparative studies of, 84
        alprazolam and, 73–75, **74, 75**
        psychological treatment and,
            101–105, 106–107
    in depression, 84
    discontinuation of, 70, 87, 88
    dosage of, 67, 70
    long-term treatment with, 70, 86
    side effects of, 67, 69, 70
3H-imipramine receptors, as
    markers, 48
*International Classification of
    Diseases* (ICD), 1, 24
    ICD-10, 6, 10, 11–12, **12**, 57
    diagnostic criteria for panic
        disorder and, 9
Interoceptive exposure, 93
    with cognitive restructuring,
        comparative outcome studies
        of, 96
Interviews, structured, diagnostic, 6
Iproniazid, 65

Irritable bowel syndrome, 19, 20
  comorbidity with, 34
Isoproterenol provocation, 47
  validity of panic disorder as
    nosological entity and, 58

Kajak-angst, 23
Kuru, 23

Laboratory studies, validity of panic
  disorder as nosological entity
  and, 58
Lactate provocation, 5, 47
  validity of panic disorder as
    nosological entity and, 58
Latah, 23
Learning theory, of etiology of panic
  disorder, 43
Life events, as precipitant, 53–54
Ligands, abnormal endogenous
  ligand theory and, 51
Limbic system, anxiety-arousal
  states and, 48
Limited symptom attacks, clinical
  and diagnostic features of, 7
Locus ceruleus, activation of
  neurons in, 49–50
Lorazepam, 71, **71,** 73
  comparative studies of, 84
    alprazolam and, 76
  dosage of, **71,** 72
  with tricyclic antidepressants, 70

Magnetic resonance imaging,
  validity of panic disorder as
  nosological entity and, 58
Maintenance therapy, 88–89
Marijuana
  heart rate increase caused by, 17
  precipitation of anxiety attacks
    by, 17
Medical care, seeking. *See*
  Help-seeking
Medical illness, 34
  cardiac. *See* Cardiovascular
    disease
  cormorbidity with, 29–30, 34–35

  mortality and, 34–35
  differential diagnosis of panic
    disorder and, **16,** 16–17
  patients presenting with
    symptoms of, 19–20
  prevalence with psychiatric
    conditions, 30
  as risk factor, 22
  worsening by arousal states, 20
Medical patients, overrepresenta-
  tion of panic attacks among, 18
Medical testing, 19
3-Methoxy-4-hydroxyphenylglycol
  (MHPG)
  cerebrospinal fluid concentration
    of, 50
  plasma concentration of, 50
Midazolam, **71**
  dosage of, **71**
Migraine headaches, 20
Minor tranquilizers, rates of use of,
  110
Misdiagnosis, 18–21
Mitral valve prolapse (MVP)
  cormorbidity with, 29
  differential diagnosis of panic
    disorder and, 16, 17
Monoamine oxidase, as marker, 48
Monoamine oxidase inhibitors
  (MAOIs), 5, 63, 65–66, 115
  as antipanic medications, **64**
  comparative studies of, 84, **85**
    tricyclic antidepressants and,
      63, 65
  drug interactions of, 65
  effectiveness in panic disorder, 27
  inhibition of activation of locus
    ceruleus by, 50
  limitations in use of, 65
  long-term treatment with, 86
  rebound with, 88
  reluctance of physicians to
    prescribe, 65
  side effects of, 66, 88
  withdrawal of, 88
Mortality, 34–36
  cardiovascular disease and, 35

Mortality *(continued)*
  suicide and, 34, 35–36
Muscle relaxation, 92
  applied relaxation compared with, 93
  comparative outcome studies of, 96, 99

National Institute of Mental Health (NIMH), 105–106
  Consensus Development Conference on the Treatment of Panic Disorder of, 1
  Panic Disorder Prevention and Public Education Program of, 19
Neurochemical theories, 49–51
Neurocirculatory asthenia, 5
Neuroendocrine markers, 48
Neurosis
  anxiety, 4–5
    Freud's use of, 4, 42
  cardiac, 4
Neurotransmitter theories, 49–51
Nocturnal panic attacks, 49
Nonfearful panic disorder, clinical and diagnostic features of, 9–10
Noradrenaline provocation, validity of panic disorder as nosological entity and, 58
Noradrenergic theory, 49–50
Norepinephrine
  cerebrospinal fluid concentration of, 50
  plasma concentration of, 50
  release of, cocaine and, 17
Norepinephrine metabolism, as marker, 48
Norepinephrine provocation, 47
Nortriptyline, 67, 69
  as antipanic medication, **64**
Nosological entity, validity of panic disorder as. *See* Validity as nosological entity

Obsessive-compulsive disorder, comorbidity with, 27

Opiates, withdrawal from, 17
Orthostatic hypotension, with tricyclic antidepressants, 69
Overdose, safety margin in, with tricyclic antidepressants, 69
Overprotection, parental, etiology of panic disorder and, 46
Oxazepam, 71, **71**
  dosage of, **71**

Panic anxiety, 6–7
  clinical manifestations of, 7, **8, 9**
  symptoms of, 7, **7**
Panic apprehension, 42
Panic attacks
  blockade of, **64,** 64–65
  clinical and diagnostic features of, 7
  Freud's description of, 4
  learning theory of, 43–44
  nocturnal, 49
  rates of use of medications in, 110
Panic-control treatments (PCTs).
  See Psychological treatment
Parahippocampal gyrus, anxiety-arousal states and, 48
Parahippocampus, blood flow in, 49
Parent(s), child-rearing attitudes and behavior of, etiology of panic disorder and, 46
Parental Bonding Instrument, 46
Pathogenesis/pathophysiology
  experimental models and biological theories of, 47–53
  animal models of anxiety and arousal states and, 48
  functional brain imaging studies and, 48–49
  neurochemical and neurotransmitter theories and, 49–51
  neuroendocrine and other biological markers and, 48
  nocturnal panic attacks and, 49
  panic disorder as variant of convulsive disorder and, 52
  provocation and challenge studies and, 47–48

working hypothesis and, 52–53
psychological and psychosocial theories of, 53–55
life events as precipitants and, 53–54
predisposing factors in adolescent and adult personality and, 54–55
Personality, predisposing factors in, 54–55
Personality disorders, comorbidity with, 28
Pharmacoepidemiology. *See* Psychopharmacological treatment, community patterns of prescription and use of antipanic medications and
Phenelzine, 65–66
as antipanic medication, **64**
comparative studies of, 84
in depression, 83
Phobia, social, 27
clomipramine in, 68
Phobic avoidance, 13
development of, learning theory of, 43
treatment of, 70, 100
therapeutic exposure in, 90–92
Pituitary, anterior, 52
Polysomnographic studies, 49
Positron-emission tomography (PET), 48–49
validity of panic disorder as nosological entity and, 58
Posttraumatic stress disorder, comorbidity with, 27
Prazepam, 71, **71**
dosage of, **71**
Precipitants, life events as, 53–54
Predisposing factors, in adolescent and adult personality, 54–55
Prescription, patterns of. *See* Psychopharmacological treatment, community patterns of prescription and use of antipanic medications and

Prevalence
of alcoholism, 37
of panic disorder, 18, 21–22
delimitation from other disorders and, 59
Programmed practice (PP), imipramine combined with, 104–105
Progressive muscle relaxation (PMR), 92
applied relaxation compared with, 93
comparative outcome studies of, 96, 99
Provocation studies, 5, 47–48, 50
validity of panic disorder as nosological entity and, 58
Psychiatric disorders. *See also specific disorders*
comorbid. *See* Comorbid panic disorder
differential diagnosis of panic disorder and, 15–16, **16**
prevalence of medical conditions with, 30
Psychoanalysis, 90
Psychoanalytic-oriented psychotherapy, 90
Psychoanalytic theories, of etiology of panic disorder, 42–43
Psychodynamic psychotherapy, 89–90
Psychodynamic theories, of etiology of panic disorder, 42–43
Psychological history, benzodiazepine withdrawal and, 80
Psychological theories, of etiology of panic disorder. *See* Etiology, psychological theories of
Psychological treatment, 89–100
in clinical practice, 115
cognitive-behavioral, 93–95
comparative studies of, 95–98
psychopharmacological treatment and, 100–103
exposure-based therapy and, 90–92

Psychological treatment *(continued)*
general considerations in, 89
long-term, 98–100
psychoanalysis and
psychoanalytic-oriented
therapy and, 89–90
psychopharmacological treatment
combined with, 103–107
relaxation training and, 92–93
supportive
in comorbid panic disorder with
agoraphobia, 96
imipramine combined with,
103–104
Psychoneurotic states, 42
Psychopharmacological treatment,
5, 61–89
benzodiazepines in. *See*
Benzodiazepine(s)
in clinical practice, 112, 114–115
community patterns of prescription and use of antipanic
medications and, 109–112
benzodiazepines and, 110
panic disorder and, 110–111
treatment considerations in
clinical practice and,
111–112
comorbid depression and,
treatment response and,
83–84
comparative studies of, 84, **85**
psychological treatment and,
100–103
historical background of, 61–65, **64**
long-term, 84–86
benzodiazepines in, 87–89
tricyclic antidepressants in,
70–71, 85–86
monoamine oxidase inhibitors in,
65–66
psychological treatment combined
with, 103–107
serotonin reuptake blocking
agents in, 81–83
therapeutic levels of dependence
and, 62

tricyclic antidepressants in. *See*
Tricyclic antidepressants
Psychophysiological studies, in
depression and panic disorder,
27
Psychosocial treatment. *See*
Cognitive-behavioral treatment
Psychotherapy
psychoanalytic-oriented, 90
psychodynamic, 89–90

Quality of life, 36–38

Rebound
with benzodiazepines, 76, 79, **80,**
87, 115
with monoamine oxidase
inhibitors, 88
with tricyclic antidepressants, 88
Relapse
following benzodiazepine
treatment, 79, **80,** 87
following tricyclic antidepressant
treatment, 70–71
Relaxation training (RT), 92–93
comparative outcome studies of,
96, 97–98
psychopharmacological
treatment and, 101–102
REM latency, shortened, in
depression and panic disorder,
27–28
Research
cross-cultural studies, 23–24
Cross-National Collaborative
Panic Study, 38, 60, 72,
73–75, **74, 75,** 83–84, 86
cross-national studies, 23–24, 38,
60, 72, 73–75, **74, 75,** 83–84,
86
directions for, 115–117
Epidemiologic Catchment Area
study, 18, 21, 24–25, 30, 37,
38
Harvard Anxiety Research
Program, 28–29, 38, 60
twin studies, 23, 40

validity of panic disorder as
nosological entity and, 60
Respiratory disorders, comorbidity
with, 34
Risk factors, 22–23
family history as, 22–23

School phobia, etiology of panic
disorder and, 45
Sedation, with benzodiazepines, 76
Sedative-hypnotics, withdrawal
from, 17
Seizure disorders, panic disorder as
variant of, 52
Selective serotonin reuptake
inhibitors (SSRIs), 81–83, 115
effectiveness in panic disorder, 27
Separation anxiety, etiology of panic
disorder and, 45
Septal region, anxiety-arousal
states and, 48
Septohippocampal region
activation of, 52–53
anxiety-arousal states and, 48
Serotonergic theory, 50
Serotonin, release of, cocaine and, 17
Serotonin metabolism, as marker, 48
Serotonin receptors
downregulation by serotonin
reuptake inhibitors, 83
downregulation by tricyclic
antidepressants, 50
Serotonin reuptake inhibitors,
81–83, 115
effectiveness in panic disorder, 27
Serotonin uptake, as marker, 48
Sex
comorbid anxiety disorder and,
agoraphobia and alcoholism
and, 29
as risk factor, 22
Sexual side effects, with benzodiazepines, 76
Sheehan Disability Scale, 37–38
Signal anxiety, 42
Sleep
panic attacks during, 49

shortened REM latency and, in
depression and panic
disorder, 27–28
Sleeping pills, rates of use of, 110
Social activities, decline in, 20–21
Social environment, benzodiazepine
withdrawal and, 80
Social morbidity, 37
Social phobia, 27
clomipramine in, 68
Sodium lactate provocation, 5, 47
validity of panic disorder as
nosological entity and, 58
"Soldier's heart," 4
Somatization, 18–19
Spouse, including in exposure-based
therapy, 91–92, 99
Stroke, risk for, in patients with
panic disorder, 30
Structured interviews, diagnostic, 6
Substance abuse. *See also*
Alcoholism
comorbidity with, 26, 77
potential of benzodiazepines for,
76–77
comorbidity and, 77
precipitation of anxiety attacks
by, 17
Suicide, deaths from, 34
Suicide attempts, 20
Supportive therapy
in comorbid panic disorder with
agoraphobia, 96
imipramine combined with,
103–104
Susto, 23

Temazepam, 71, **71**
dosage of, **71**
Thalamus, 52
Tranquilizers
benzodiazepine. *See* Benzodiaze-
pine(s)
minor, rates of use of, 110
Transmission mode, 41
Tranylcypromine, 65
as antipanic medication, **64**

Tranylcypromine *(continued)*
comparative studies of, 84
side effects of, 66
Trazodone, 27
Treatment, 61–108
in clinical practice, 111–112
cognitive-behavioral. *See*
Cognitive-behavioral
treatment
general considerations in, 61
long-term, 31
newer, 31–32, **32, 33**
psychological. *See* Psychological
treatment
psychopharmacological. *See*
Psychopharmacological
treatment; *specific drugs and
drug classes*
short-term, 31
undertreatment and, 18–19, 20–21
Triazolam, 71, **71**
dosage of, **71**
Tricyclic antidepressants (TCAs), 5,
64, 66–71, 115. *See also specific
drugs*
adverse effects of, 69–70
as antipanic medications, **64**
benzodiazepines with, 70
clinical issues with, 70
comparative studies of, 84, **85**
monoamine oxidase inhibitors
and, 63, 65
discontinuation of, 70
dosage of, 70–71
maintenance, 70
downregulation of 5-HT
autoreceptors by, 50
effectiveness in panic disorder, 27
general considerations with, 66
inhibition of activation of locus
ceruleus by, 50
long-term treatment with, 85–86
dose during, 70–71
psychological therapy combined
with, 105

psychopharmacological treatment
response to, 83–84
rebound and, 88
relapse following treatment with,
70–71
side effects of, 67, 68, 69, 70, 88
withdrawal of, 88
Twin studies, 23, 40
validity of panic disorder as
nosological entity and, 60

Uncomplicated panic disorder, 24–25
suicide risk and, 35
Undertreatment, 18–19, 20–21

Validity as nosological entity, 57–60
clinical description and, 57, 58
delimitation from other disorders,
57, 59
family and twin studies and, 57,
60
follow-up studies and, 57, 60
laboratory studies and, 57, 58

Weight gain
with benzodiazepines, 88
with tricyclic antidepressants, 69
Withdrawal symptoms, 17
with benzodiazepines, 76, 78, **79,**
115
factors influencing, 77–81, **81**
with monoamine oxidase
inhibitors, 88
with opiates, 17
sedative-hypnotics and, 17
with tricyclic antidepressants, 88
World Psychiatric Association, Task
Force on Panic Anxiety and Its
Treatments of, 1

Yohimbine provocation, 5, 47, 50
validity of panic disorder as
nosological entity and, 58

Zimelidine, 81